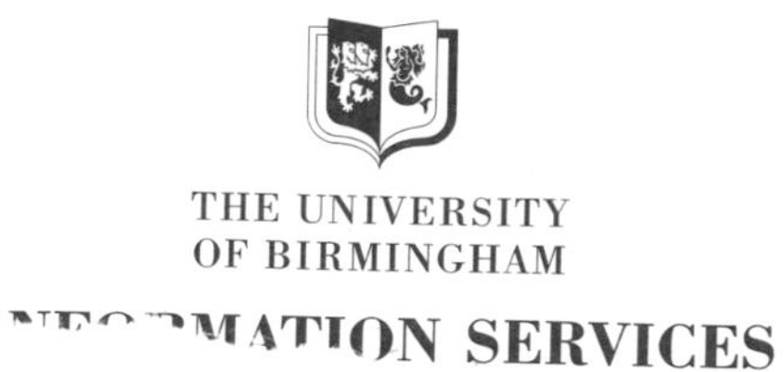

Routine Blood Results Explained

Forthcoming titles from M&K Publishing

2006

Issues in Heart Failure Nursing
ISBN 978 1-905539-00-2 – May 2006

Self Assessment in –
Musculoskeletal trauma imaging of appendicular skeleton
ISBN 978 1-905539-13-4 – May 2006

Improving Patient Outcomes: a guide for Ward Managers
ISBN 978 -1-905539-06-1 – May 2006

The ECG Workbook
ISBN 978-1-905539-14-7 – June 2006

Emergency Management for Nurses
ISBN 978 1-905539-05-3 – June 2006

Nurse Facilitated Hospital Discharge
ISBN 978 -1-905539-12-6 – July 2006

The Advanced Respiratory Practitioner:
a practical & theoretical guide for Nurses & AHPs
ISBN 978-1-905539-10-9 – September 2006

Pre-Operative Assessment and Perioperative Management
ISBN 978 1-905539-02-9 – September 2006

Pre-teen and Teenage Pregnancy: a 21st century reality
ISBN 978 1-905539-11-8 – December 2006

2007

Nurse Consultancy
ISBN 978-1-905539-09-3 – February 2007

Ophthalmic Assessment
ISBN 978 1-905539-08-6 – March 2007

Managing Emotions in Women's Health
ISBN 978 1-905539-07-X – April 2007

Routine Blood Results Explained

Dr Andrew Blann
PhD FRCPath

Consultant Clinical Scientist
and Honorary Senior Lecturer in Medicine

Haemostasis, Thrombosis and Vascular Biology Unit
University Department of Medicine
City Hospital, Dudley Road
Birmingham B18 7QH

Routine Blood Results Explained
Dr Andrew Blann PhD FRCPath

ISBN: 1-905539-01-0

First published 2006

24194263

All rights reserved. No part of this publication may be reproduced, stored in a retrieval system, or transmitted in any form or by any means, electronic, mechanical, photocopying, recording or otherwise, without either the prior permission of the publishers or a licence permitting restricted copying in the United Kingdom issued by the Copyright Licensing Agency, 90 Tottenham Court Road, London, W1T 4LP. Permissions may be sought directly from M&K Publishing, phone: 01768 773030, fax: 01768 781099 or email: publishing@mkupdate.co.uk
Any person who does any unauthorised act in relation to this publication may be liable to criminal prosecution and civil claims for damages.

British Library Catalogue in Publication Data
A catalogue record for this book is available from the British Library

Notice:
Clinical practice and medical knowledge constantly evolve. Standard safety precautions must be followed, but, as knowledge is broadened by research, changes in practice, treatment and drug therapy may become necessary or appropriate. Readers must check the most current product information provided by the manufacturer of each drug to be administered and verify the dosages and correct administration, as well as contraindications. It is the responsibility of the practitioner, utilising the experience and knowledge of the patient, to determine dosages and the best treatment for each individual patient. Neither the publisher nor the authors assume any liability for any injury and/or damage to persons or property arising from this publication.

The Publisher

To contact M&K Publishing write to:
M&K Update Ltd · The Old Bakery · St. John's Street
Keswick · Cumbria CA12 5AS

Tel: 01768 773030 · Fax: 01768 781099
publishing@mkupdate.co.uk
www.mkupdate.co.uk

Designed & typeset in 10pt Usherwood Book by Mary Blood
Printed by Gloss Image Ltd, Dewsbury

. . . it is estimated that the data received by Clinicians from Medical Laboratories constitutes 70–80 % of the information they rely on to make major medical decisions . . .

The Biomedical Scientist 2005, 49:38

Dedication

To Burt and Dorcas, for all their love.

To Edward, Eleanor and Rosie, with all my love.

Contents

Preface

The objective of this slim volume is to provide help in understanding and interpreting the majority of the normal blood results found in most NHS Hospitals. The text, based on the routine blood report forms sent out from Pathology Departments, has evolved from lecture notes given to various Health Care Professionals (Nurses, Phlebotomists, Pharmacists, Radiographers, Physiotherapists etc.) attending day-long courses on exactly these topics.

Fortunately, the vast majority of routine blood tests, certainly in routine, emergency and critical care medicine, fall easily into one of two groups – haematology and biochemistry. The layout of the volume will therefore follow that pattern. Each of the two major sections breaks down into individual Chapters and concludes with a dedicated example. Furthermore, each of the two major sections ends with case studies designed to test the ability of the reader to assess what they have learned.

An additional objective is to keep the material simple and focused. Thus, the reader seeking a comprehensive in-depth explanation of a wide number of tests and their exact relationship to various clinical diseases will be disappointed. However, it is impossible to fully understand pathology without a sure grounding in physiology. Hence there will be an adequate and clear explanation of those aspects of the body that are necessary to understand a particular test and its associated problems. Examples are provided that will illustrate particular points; it must be stressed that these are not exact and perfect case reports, merely aids in understanding the concepts developed in the text.

Focusing on 'routine' blood tests therefore, by definition, excludes tests less frequently reported. In this volume, tests that will be absent from the general discussion are, for example, platelet volume, red cell mass, magnesium, and reproductive hormones. These omissions are not indicative of lack of importance, merely lack of regular requesting. The emphasis is also on the adult, so that paediatric tests (by and large) will not be mentioned.

The 'normal' range

In trying to define ill-health, we generally use good health as a comparator. Thus a healthy person can be expected to have a certain healthy blood result profile. However, these values are sometimes not well established and are subject to change.

Furthermore, there are many normal (healthy) people whose blood result may not be in the normal range – this does not necessarily mean they are ill. Therefore the concept of being 'normal' may as well be 'desirable'. So you could use a 'reference' range, or perhaps a 'target' range. However, for the purposes of this volume, the normal range will be cited.

Haematology and biochemistry are very quantitative sciences. Consequently, the normal range is important. The precise definition of the normal range in use at a particular hospital is crucial and is not transferable to another hospital. This may be because of small differences in the technical manner in which tests are derived. Furthermore, normal ranges may well (or actually should) reflect the local population that the hospital serves, and this is important as different catchment populations may well vary considerably, especially in ethnicity.

It is also becoming the case that results will be provided with a normal range suitable for the demography of the particular patient, i.e. a male normal range for blood from a man, a paediatric normal range for an infant etc. Therefore, care must be taken when comparing samples and normal ranges. In the future it can be predicted that an age-specific and race-specific normal range may also be produced.

In clinical blood science (as haematology and biochemistry are merging or evolving into) the numbers mean something. Many will seek guidance from, and will base treatment on, these results. One of the first questions is therefore 'is the result acceptable?' This in turn begs the question of acceptability, which in many cases boils down to the normal range, presumably derived from normal, i.e. healthy, individuals. However, merely having a result a fraction outside the normal range does not necessarily imply a serious pathology. Conversely, a result very far from the normal range carries with it an implication of a problem. Several tests, as well as clinical signs, history, etc. are needed to be sure of a particular diagnosis.

The normal ranges cited in Appendices 1 and 2 (pages 125 and 126) are for the use of this book alone. They are not transferable to your own hospital or practice, as you may have a different normal range. This is entirely normal practice.

Acknowledgments
With thanks to my colleagues Alan Walls, Mike Yegwart and Sukhjinder Marwah.
The photographs of warfarin-induced skin necrosis are with the kind permission of Stephan Moll, Department of Medicine, University of North Carolina, USA *British Journal of Haematology* 2004, 126: 628

Abbreviations

ALL	Acute lymphocyte or lymphoblastic leukaemia
AML	Acute myeloid leukaemia
APTT	Activated partial thromboplastin time
ARF	Acute renal failure
CAOD	Chronic obstructive airways disease
CGL	Chronic granulocytic leukaemia
CK	Creatine kinase
CLL	Chronic lymphocytes leukaemia
CRF	Chronic renal failure
CRP	C-reactive protein
DKA	Diabetic ketoacidosis (DKA)
DVT	Deep vein thrombosis
ECG	Electrocardiogram
EDTA	Ethylene diamine tetra-acetic acid
ESR	Erythrocyte sedimentation rate
FBC	Full blood count
GFR	Glomerular filtration rate
Hct	Haematocrit
Hb	Haemoglobin
HbA1c	Glycosylated haemoglobin
HDL-cholesterol	High density lipoprotein cholesterol
INR	International normalised ratio
LDL-cholesterol	Low density lipoprotein cholesterol
LFTs	Liver function tests
LMWH	Low molecular weight heparin
MCH	Mean cell haemoglobin
MCHC	Mean cell haemoglobin concentration
MCV	Mean cell volume
OGTT	Oral glucose tolerance test
PTH	Parathyroid hormone
PSA	Prostate specific antigen
PT	Prothrombin time
PTT	Partial thromboplastin time
PE	Pulmonary embolus
RBCC/RCC	Red blood cell count/red cell count
T4	Thyroxine
TSH	Thyroid stimulating hormone
U&E	Urea and electrolytes
WBCC/WCC	White blood cell count/white cell count

Part 1

Haematology

Haematology:
Objectives and Scope

Objectives and scope

These are listed in Table 1. The basic purpose of the Haematology Laboratory is to provide assistance in the diagnosis, monitoring and treatment of patients. In order to do this, the components of the blood are analysed, almost always in custom-designed equipment. It is taken as understood that all blood tubes and forms must be fully labelled by those taking the blood in order to minimise the risk of (possibly fatal) error. Indeed, the laboratory will be well within its rights to decline to test a sample that is incorrectly or inadequately labelled.

There are three basic blood tubes that are used in the haematology laboratory. A full blood count (FBC) is performed on blood that is anticoagulated with the potassium salt of ethylene diamine tetra-acetic acid (EDTA). Coagulation tests are invariably done on plasma that is obtained from whole blood anticoagulated with sodium citrate. The erythrocyte sedimentation rate (ESR) is assessed on blood that is held within its own dedicated glass tube: blood clotting in this tube is also prevented by sodium citrate.

Testing can only be performed on blood that is collected in the correct tube. Failure to do so will, at best, result in a polite phone call from the lab explaining the problem and its remedy. At worse, a report will be returned a day or so later with a comment such as 'inappropriate blood sample received, please repeat'. Fortunately, many blood tubes have different coloured tops to help this process and minimise errors.

In some Pathology Departments, certain tests are done in the Haematology Laboratory, whilst in other hospitals, the same test may be performed in the Biochemistry Laboratory. Examples of this include iron studies, C-reactive protein (CRP), and testing for vitamin B_{12} and serum folate. However, these tests are done on serum obtained from whole blood that has not been anticoagulated. The reader is referred to their own Pathology Service for the correct tube for the test and the destination of these requests.

Overall, our colleagues in the Pathology Department, regardless of discipline, would far rather set the position clear in a phone call than go through the bother of phoning back that a fresh sample in the correct tube must be obtained. If in doubt – PHONE !!

A note on units

A note on units. In the real world, of course, results are almost unanimously described as the numbers alone (e.g. haemoglobin 12.5) instead of the more correct way where the result is described with its unit (i.e. 12.5 g/L). This shorthand is (almost) universally accepted, and generally makes life considerable easier. It matters not so much that the correct unit of the average size of a red blood cell is described fully, for example, as 112 fL, or in shorthand simply as 112, but it does matter that the particular cell is much larger than can be expected in complete health, implying ill-health.

Fortunately, Haematology can be divided very easily into four different areas. These are the red blood cell, the white blood cell, coagulation and blood transfusion. The most important aspects of each of these are, in turn, anaemia, infection and neoplasia, thrombosis and haemorrhage, and a transfusion reaction, respectively. Finally, it would be good if the reader is able to translate these concepts into 'real-life' interpretation, such as the implications of a haemoglobin count of 8.4 g/dL, with or without a white blood cell count of 15 x 10^9/L, the possible problems and benefits of INR of 4.0, and the consequences of an incompatible blood transfusion.

The forms that follow (Figure 1) are those produced by the author's laboratory for the end user (i.e. the requesting practitioner) and will generally end up in the patient's notes (in this case note that the patient is the author!). Apart from the usual demographic details (age, sex, hospital number, ward, Consultant etc.), the report offers (from left to right) a column of abbreviations (particular tests), a column of numbers (the result), another column of numbers and letters (units), and yet another column of numbers (the [male] normal or target range).

The top form is the full blood count, the lower form is the coagulation profile.

The main objective of this section of the book is to explain to you what all this means.

Figure 1 Haematology Report Form

Sandwell and West Birmingham Hospitals NHS Trust — Haematology, City Hospital

Surname BLANN
Forename Andrew
D.O.B. 11.08.54
NHS No. *
Address
Unit No.
Consultant/GP Not Given
Lab No. C.050230313 C
ASCOT CLINIC
ASCOT STUDY

Clinical Details

HB	14.6	g/dL	(13.3 – 16.7)
MCV	93.0	fL	(80.0 – 98.0)
WBC	6.8	10^9/L	(3.7 – 9.5)
PLT	288	10^9/L	(143 – 400)
RBC	4.61	10^12/L	(4.32 – 5.66)
HCT	42.8	%	(39.0 – 50.0)
MCH	31.8	pg	(27.3 – 32.6)
MCHC	34.2	g/dL	(31.6 – 34.9)
NEUT	4.57	10^9/L	(1.70 – 6.10)
LYMPH	1.67	10^9/L	(1.00 – 3.20)
MONO	0.39	10^9/L	(0.20 – 0.60)
EOS	0.07	10^9/L	(0.03 – 0.46)
BASO	* 0.01	10^9/L	(0.02 – 0.09)

HY	0.2	%	(0.0 – 7.9)

Tests FBC, %HY
Check Clinician
Date received 12.11.05
Date reported 12.11.05

Sandwell and West Birmingham Hospitals NHS Trust — Haematology, City Hospital

Surname BLANN
Forename Andrew
D.O.B. 11.08.54
NHS No. *
Address
Unit No.
Consultant/GP Not Given
Lab No. C.05.0230313.C
ASCOT CLINIC
ASCOT STUDY

Clinical Details

PT	13	secs	(11-14)
INR	1.1		
PTT	28	secs	(24-34)
PTT Ratio	1.0		
Fib	2.9	g/L	(1.5-4.0)

Tests APTT, FIB, PT
Check Clinician
Date received 12.11.05
Date reported 12.11.05

Table 1
Learning Objectives – Haematology

Learning objectives – haematology

Having completed these notes in a satisfactory manner, the reader will. . .

1. Appreciate the importance of different anticoagulants and glass tubes for the different blood tests requested: EDTA (full blood count) and sodium citrate (coagulation). ESR has its own special tube. The Blood Bank generally needs a sample of clotted blood or blood taken into EDTA.

2. Recognise the four major areas of interest, i.e.
- The red blood cell
- The white blood cell
- Coagulation
- Blood transfusion

3. Describe major problems associated with each of these three areas, e.g., respectively
- Anaemia
- Infection/neoplasia
- Thrombosis/haemorrhage
- An incompatible blood transfusion

4. Interpret simple haematological results, e.g.
- A haemoglobin of 8.4 g/L
- A white cell count of 15 x 10^9/L
- A prothrombin time of 25 seconds.

5. Understand the importance of the Haematology Laboratory

Chapter 1

The Red Blood Cell

Key words:

Haemoglobin (Hb)
Red blood cell count (RBCC)
Haematocrit (Hct)
Red cell indices:
- Mean cell volume (MCV)
- Mean cell haemoglobin (MCH)
- Mean cell haemoglobin concentration (MCHC)

Erythrocyte sedimentation rate (ESR).

Plasma viscosity (n.b. not strictly to do with the red blood cell)

Key pathological expressions:

Anaemia
Polycythaemia
Thalassaemia
Sickle cell disease

An explanation of terms:

Haemoglobin

Haemoglobin (Hb): Normal/reference range in men 13.3 to 16.7 g/dL, in women 11.8 to 14.8 g/dL

Haemoglobin is undoubtedly the index most frequently referred to in clinical haematology. It is a protein designed to carry oxygen from the lungs to the tissues, where the oxygen is given up to participate in respiration. The normal range varies between the sexes. Lower levels in menstruating women seem obvious, but in post-menopausal women levels are still lower than age-matched men as the latter produce testosterone to stimulate red cell production.

Red blood cell count

The red blood cell count (RBCC): Normal range in men 4.32 to 5.66 x 10^{12}/L, in women 3.88 to 4.99 x 10^{12}/L

Haemoglobin is carried in the blood in red blood cells. These are unusual as they lack a nucleus, thus providing additional flexibility to penetrate the smallest capillaries. They are the most abundant cell in the blood, are often called erythrocytes, and numbers can also vary between the sexes.

Haematocrit

Haematocrit (Hct): Normal range in men 39 to 50%, in women, 36 to 44%

This index expresses that proportion, as a decimal or as a percentage, of whole blood that is taken up by all the blood cells. Since there are approximately a thousand more red blood cells per unit volume than both white blood cells and (tiny) platelets, the red cells make up the major proportion of the haematocrit. Consequently, at the practical level, it provides an idea of the proportion of red blood cells that makes up the whole blood pool.

Red blood cell indices

The red blood cell indices

These are:

- Mean cell volume (MCV, 80–98 fL) is the size of the average (mean) red blood cell. Note the stress is on 'average', as each index is the mean of millions of individual cells.
- Mean cell haemoglobin (MCH, normal range 27.3–32.6 pg), as the name implies, simply reports the average amount (mass) of haemoglobin in the average cell. It does not take into account the size of the cell.
- Mean cell haemoglobin concentration (MCHC, 31.6–34.9 pg/dL) is the average concentration of haemoglobin inside the average size cell.

Error may easily be introduced as, for example, an MCV of, shall we say, 90 fL, may arise from cells with very diverse size, ranging from 70 to 110. Cells of such diverse size must imply one or more pathological process (such as alcoholism). But the same MCV of 90 may also be the sum of a very well regulated population of cells that vary from, in this example, 87 to 93. For this reason, MCV is probably the most useful of the three indices, especially in investigating different types of anaemia, as we shall see.

Because several of the red cell values are mathematically derived from some of the others, it is entirely possible for any one of them to be outside the normal range whilst the other five are apparently normal. Thus one must consider all six red cell indices (and possibly some others) together to obtain a full picture. In the author's laboratory, the Bayer Advia 120 provides Hb, RBCC and MCV directly from the blood provided to it, then (simply speaking) calculates the Hct from the RBCC times the MCV, the MCH by the Hb divided by the RBCC, and the MCHC by the Hb divided by the Hct, with adjustments (e.g. times or divide by 10 or 100).

ESR

Erythrocyte sedimentation rate (ESR): Normally <10 mm/hour

The ESR is also a global score of physical aspects of the blood, and is simple to understand. The result is obtained by allowing a thin column of blood to settle down under the influence of gravity. As it does so, the red blood cells will separate from the plasma, so that after an hour, a band of clear plasma will sit atop the red blood cells. The fall in the level of the red blood cells is then recorded as mm/hour. The effects of platelets and white blood cells are minimal and are ignored. It is therefore unique in requiring no sophisticated machinery and few technical skills.

An increased ESR can be caused by many factors, including cancer, anaemia, inflammation, rheumatoid arthritis, multiple myeloma and tuberculosis. It is increased soon after myocardial infarction, and is also heavily influenced by plasma proteins.

Some laboratories have a more liberal normal range, e.g. <20 mm/hour, especially in the elderly.

Plasma viscosity

Plasma viscosity: Normal range 1.5 to 1.75 mPa

Plasma viscosity does not really have much to do with red blood cells, but is in this Chapter purely for convenience. It is most often measured in the Haematology Laboratory.

This index provides an idea of how thick or thin the plasma has become – whether or not it is thinner, and more like water (tending towards a low result of less than 1.5), or thicker and more like treacle (tending towards a high result, over 1.72). Viscosity records a global property of the plasma, not individual molecules. Indeed, the molecules that make up the major component of viscosity include fibrinogen, albumin and some proteins involved in clotting. There is also a relationship between plasma viscosity and total plasma protein concentration, and often with the haematocrit (Hct) and the amount of water in the blood.

What are red cells for ?

Red cells

The answer to this question is easy: to carry oxygen. The oxygen-carrying capacity of the blood is a function not only of the amount of haemoglobin in each cell, but also the number of red blood cells and, to a lesser extent, the haematocrit. In this way someone with a low MCH but a high RBCC may well have the same oxygen-carrying capacity as someone else with a higher MCH but a lower RBCC. Red cells can also contribute to clotting.

Haemoglobin, RBCC, Hct and the three red cell indices of MCV, MCH and MCHC are requested to obtain a view of the individual's oxygen carrying capacity. When an individual is having difficulty performing their most basic physiological and lifestyle demands, they could be anaemic. Some authorities will define anaemia as a level of haemoglobin below a certain level. However, a haemoglobin level of, say, 11.5 g/dL may well be perfectly adequate for an elderly person with few physiological requirements and a relatively quite life. However, the same haemoglobin level in a younger person with a very active lifestyle, perhaps including sports, will be inadequate. Thus the medical state of the individual as a whole person should be considered, not merely an arbitrary number at which one acts. An alternative view of anaemia may be the level at which concern arises, and at which further investigations are considered. Certainly, anaemia should not be seen merely as that level that automatically requires a blood transfusion, a therapy that many consider should be reserved only for life-saving situations (see Chapter 4).

The aetiology and classification of anaemia

Anaemia

Anaemia may be classified in many ways (Table 2).

Since red blood cells are produced in the bone marrow, infiltration of this tissue by cancer or other cells will inevitably lead to a reduction in the production of the red cells, thus anaemia. Anaemia is also a fundamental aspect of aplastic anaemia, where the other functions of the bone marrow (i.e. the production of platelets and normal white blood cells) are also depressed. As we shall see, this is also the case in leukaemia, where many abnormal white blood cells make up the tumour. Our present view of medicine offers various drugs in an attempt to solve many problems. However, few, if any, drugs are free of undesirable side effects, and one can be bone marrow suppression. Thus many drugs will call for frequent monitoring to check for the development of, for example, low levels of red blood cells.

Classification of anaemia

Table 2
A Simple Classification of Anaemia

1. Depressed red blood cell production from the bone marrow
   - Due to infiltrating cancer (e.g. leukaemia, or secondaries from elsewhere)
   - Due to total marrow shut down (e.g. aplastic anaemia, or due to drugs)

2. Diet deficiency
   - Iron
   - Vitamins B_{12} and folate
   - Plasma proteins (for building essential carriage and storage molecules)

3. Loss of mature red blood cells
   - Drugs
   - Fevers, infections
   - Auto-immunity
   - Acute or chronic bleeding

4. Haemoglobinopathy
   - Sickle cell disease
   - Thalassaemia

Poor nutrition will also result in anaemia, and a diet lacking essential factors such as iron, vitamin B_{12} or folate are good examples. However, the diet itself may be adequate, but other factors may cause anaemia, such as failure to produce special proteins to aid the passage of the minerals and vitamins across the gut wall and into the blood (i.e. malabsorption).

Problems with other organs may also contribute to anaemia. Chronic liver disease may be a factor in anaemia as it produces molecules that store and others that transport essential iron and vitamins around the body (e.g. the specialised protein transferrin for carrying iron). Intestinal disease or malabsorption may also lead to anaemia, as the ability to absorb essential minerals and vitamins will be impaired. The kidney produces a hormone, erythropoietin, to stimulate the bone marrow to produce red blood cells. Thus chronic renal failure may contribute to an anaemia.

Haemolytic anaemia is the bursting, destruction, or inappropriate break-up of red blood cells. Possible mechanisms for this include physical destruction by, for example, a poorly functioning mechanical heart valve, prolonged heavy exercise, or long marches undertaken by the armed forces. Certain individuals are sensitive to drugs (such as antibiotics) that stick onto the surface of red blood cells and render them more susceptible to attack and degradation. High fever may also destroy red blood cells, as will infections such as malaria. Autoimmune haemolytic anaemia occurs when antibodies are produced which (erroneously) bind to red blood cells. This will make the cell a target of the immune system and will lead to their elimination, often in the spleen.

Red blood cells may be lost by an acute or chronic bleed. The former may include bleeding after surgery, heavy menstrual bleeding, or bleeding by a ruptured blood vessel that may leak into the intestines. If this process is occult, or prolonged, it may lead to a chronic state of blood loss. In these types of anaemia, there is nothing intrinsically wrong with the blood cells themselves.

The most common congenital haemoglobinopathies are sickle cell disease and thalassaemia, genetic conditions characterised by qualitative changes in the haemoglobin molecule that severely reduce its ability to transport oxygen. These cells also have a shorter lifespan than cells carrying normal haemoglobin, and both conditions are associated with a variety of clinical conditions such as jaundice and skin ulcers.

There are, of course, many more possible types of anaemia. The above simply lists major causes.

Size matters!

The three red cell indices of MCH, MCHC and MCV can also be used to further classify anaemia. For example, in the anaemia that follows problems with vitamin B_{12}, the red blood cells are larger than normal (e.g. greater than 98 fL), and are said to be *macrocytes*, thus giving *macrocytic anaemia*. Conversely, some haemoglobinopathies and iron deficient states often lead to *microcytic anaemia* because the red blood cells are small (e.g. less than 80 fL) and are called *microcytes*. MCH and MCHC will also be altered in accord, and this may have clinical implications. Finally, a *normocytic anaemia* may be associated with a normal sized red blood cell (a *normocyte*, between 80 and 98 fL) but a lower overall haemoglobin level.

A prime reason for a normocytic anaemia will be the sudden loss of a large number of (healthy) red blood cells, perhaps by an accident, through a perforated duodenal ulcer, or bleeding gastrointestinal cancer. Here, there is nothing intrinsically wrong with the red cells themselves, the anaemia follows from another problem. Treatment therefore follows aetiology: more iron in the diet will not help a malabsorption anaemia but intravenous iron may increase the haemoglobin level.

Figure 2 **Red cell size**

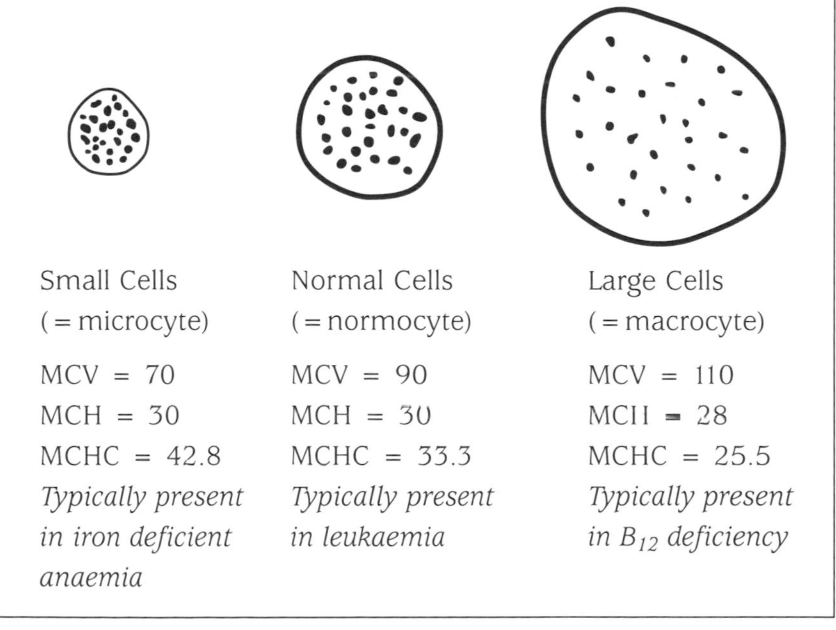

This simply illustrates how the three red cell indices can vary – the MCH is roughly the same in each case, but with different MCVs, then the MCHC is also different. This may well be important in certain conditions.

A Cautionary Tale – I

In the past there was great debate as to the definition of anaemia, such as the haemoglobin count being less than a pre-defined level of 8, 9, 10 or even (marginally) below the normal range. Consider this case report.

The case is a woman in her 30s with homozygous sickle cell disease. She was a fully-trained pharmacist, had worked full-time, had one uneventful and successful pregnancy, and had never received a blood transfusion. When she was last seen in her Clinic in Jamaica her haemoglobin was 3.9. Was she anaemic?

In 1997 she emigrated to the USA, and two years later was seen routinely by her family doctor who found a haemoglobin result of 3.8. Again – was she anaemic? Her family doctor and colleagues apparently believed so, and she was transfused with six units of blood within 24 hours.This increased her haematocrit from 11% to 31%, but also increased her systolic and diastolic blood pressures by 30 mm Hg each. Nine hours after the last transfusion she reported a headache, subsequently developed cerebral haemorrhage, and later died.

I will not discuss this case further as, I believe, it is self-explanatory. However, the report concludes with '. . . the award of US$11.5 million recommended by the jury in this case could have been avoided'. Other comments on blood transfusion follow in Chapter 4.

Source: Serjeant, G. Blood transfusion in sickle cell disease: a cautionary tale. *Lancet* 2003, 361: 1659–60.

Increased levels of red cell indices

Ideally, the healthy body tightly regulates the numbers and quality of the various aspects of the red blood cells. However, in rare instances, high levels are reported.

Polycythaemia is an excess overall red cell mass and is generally associated with a high haemoglobin, RBCC and haematocrit. This condition may arise from a rare kind of malignancy or over-activity of the bone marrow (i.e. polycythaemia ruba vera), but more generally results from the response of the bone marrow to reduced levels of oxygen. This is understandable in those people living at a very high altitude (up mountains) where the air is very thin and of low oxygen content, but in the UK, this cannot be the case. The most common form of polycythaemia is reactive to hypoxia, and the most common form of this is an unhealthy lifestyle with heavy smoking. A contributing factor is that tobacco smoke contains carbon monoxide, which binds irreversibly to haemoglobin and prevents it carrying oxygen, leading to poor oxygen carrying capacity and thus a pseudo-anaemia. The bone marrow responds by producing high numbers of excess red blood cells in an attempt to improve (restore) oxygen-carrying capacity. Consequently, this places an extra strain on the heart and circulation.

Possibly for the same reason (response to hypoxia), an increased red blood cell count can be seen in chronic anaemia such as thalassaemia.

Summary of red blood cells

Summary

- Haemoglobin (Hb) is the key index used to investigate anaemia.
- To aid precise diagnosis, the causes of the anaemia, and directions for treatment, RBCC, Hct and MCV are frequently referred to.
- Often less useful, but occasionally very enlightening, are MCH and MCHC.
- ESR and plasma viscosity are non-specific markers: an abnormal result could reflect a variety of different pathologies.

Case Study 1

A 20-year old female has recently moved, with her family, to this country from the Far East. Following a few weeks' acclimatisation and recovery from jet lag, it became clear to her family that she was consistently tired and lethargic, more so than her siblings, but had no symptoms of infection (e.g. a fever). Blood results were as follows.

Haemoglobin	10.5 g/dL,	**RBCC**	6.0 x 10^{12}/L
MCH	17.5 pg	**MCV**	55 fL
MCHC	31.8 pg/dL	**Hct**	33%
ESR	4 mm/hour	**Plasma viscosity**	1.62 mPa

See page 125 for the normal ranges of these indices, find out which are abnormal, and then make your interpretation.

Interpretation

The abnormal results are reduced haemoglobin, MCV, MCH, MCHC and Hct, with raised a red cell count. The ESR and plasma viscosity are within the normal range. With a haemoglobin level below the bottom of the normal range of 11.8 for a young woman, and the symptoms, we would have little difficulty in describing her result as concerning, and would therefore probably label her as anaemic. Very heavy menstrual periods may possibly produce this picture, but as the red blood cells are not simply small (i.e. MCV <80), but are very small (<60), we would have no hesitation in describing a microcytic anaemia, not an anaemia due to simple blood loss by itself. High numbers of red blood cells may well be a response to the oxygen-carrying problem.

The most common reasons for microcytic anaemia are iron deficiency, sickle cell disease and thalassaemia. Iron status can be easily tested for, and a test for sickle cell disease is also very simple to perform. However, both types of haemoglobinopathies are ultimately diagnosed by another test (chromatography, HPLC). Thus with a normal iron profile and negative sickle test, thalassaemia would seem to be an appropriate diagnosis.

Chapter 2

The White Blood Cell

Key words:

White blood cell count (WBCC)
The differential
Neutrophils
Lymphocytes
Monocytes
Eosinophils
Basophils
Blasts/atypical cells.

Key pathological expressions:

Leukocytosis and leukopenia
Leukaemia
Lymphoma and myeloma
Inflammation and immunity
Phagocytosis

An explanation of terms:

White blood cell count

White blood cell count:
Normal range from 3.7 to 9.5 x 10^9/L
White blood cells, or leukocytes, are collectively responsible for defending us from attack by micro-organisms such as viruses, bacteria and parasites, when raised levels of these cells can be expected. However, increased numbers may also be present in a number of conditions such as rheumatoid arthritis and cancer, and also after surgery and, as we shall see in detail, in leukaemia. Haematologists currently recognise five different types of white blood cells that can be found in the (normal) blood. The WBCC differential reports the numbers or proportions of these cells,

which are neutrophils, lymphocytes, monocytes, eosinophils and basophils. There are also a few cells called blasts, or atypical cells.

The WBCC differential

The WBCC differential

This is the proportion of the different types of leukocytes. A typical report may be neutrophils 70%, lymphocytes 20%, monocytes 7%, eosinophils 2% and basophils <1% (see the normal range, page 125). However, in pathology, these proportions will be altered. The differential may also be reported as the absolute number of each type of cell. So if the WBCC is 7.5 x 10^9/L, then the number of lymphocytes will be 1.5 x 10^9/L if the differential, as above, is 20%. However, in a reaction to a virus, the lymphocyte count may rise four-fold, to, for example, 6 x 10^9/L. If all the other leukocytes remain the same, then total WBCC will have increased to 12 x 10^9/L, which is outside the normal range, and the proportion of lymphocytes will have increased to 50%, also above the normal range.

Figure 3 **An Illustration of White Blood Cells**

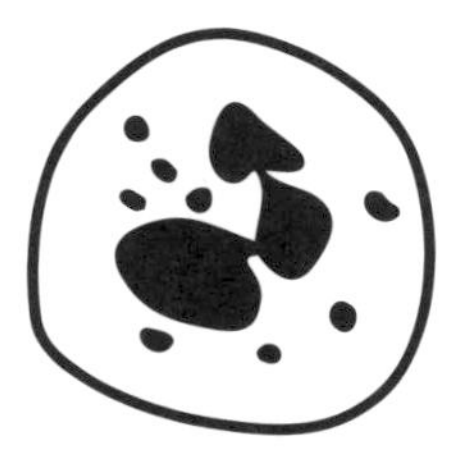

Neutrophils (normally 40 to 75% of the WBCC)

Some authorities may describe these cells, which are the most common leukocytes, as polymorphonuclear leukocytes (i.e. many different [irregular] shapes, usually three to five), granulocytes (i.e. with granules in the cytoplasm), or simply as polymorphs. However, basophils and eosinophils also have an irregular nucleus and have granules, so that others may consider these cells also to be polymorphs and granulocytes.

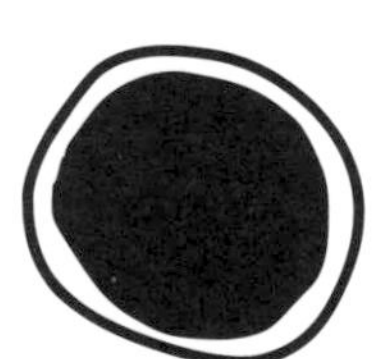

Lymphocytes (normally 20 to 45% of the WBCC)

The second most common group of leukocytes, lymphocytes differ principally from neutrophils by the structure of their nucleus, which is round and regular in contrast to the neutrophil's numerous irregular shapes. These cells are also normally smaller than neutrophils, and don't have granules.

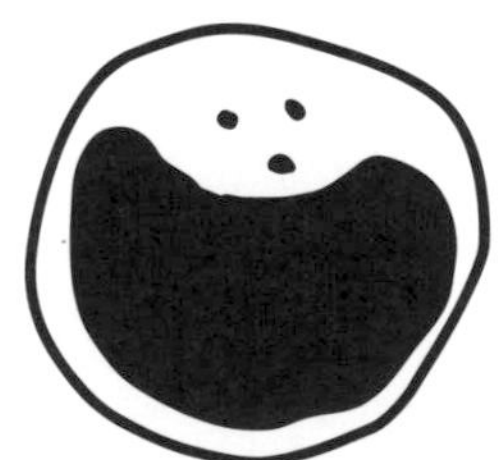

Monocytes (normally 2 to 10% of the WBCC)

These cells often resemble lymphocytes as they also have a round, regular nucleus. However, the nucleus of most monocytes does not take up as much of the cell, maybe up to 80%, whereas the lymphocyte nucleus frequently occupies over 95% of the cells. Monocytes are also larger than lymphocytes. It is often suggested that many monocytes are only temporarily in the blood on their way to the tissues where they reside.

Eosinophils

Eosinophils (normally 1 to 6% of the WBCC)
These cells are so-called because of the reddish colour, due to the chemical make up of their granules. The nucleus is of composed of just two parts, linked together by a small thread.

Basophils

Basophils (normally less than 1% of the WBCC)
The least frequent of the normal leukocytes, basophils contain numerous granules that take up different dyes, and so appear as black or dark blue. They resemble eosinophils in size and nuclear shape, but are not red.

Blasts/ atypical cells

Blasts/atypical cells: (normally less than 1% of the WBCC)
There will generally be great agreement amongst haematologists about definitions of the five major sub-types of white blood cells. However, occasionally the odd cell appears in the blood that defies this simple classification. Such cells, often with unusual characteristics, may be described as blasts or atypical cells.

However, in certain clear disease, as will be outlined below, increased number of blasts carry pathological implications, some of which are profound. An example of this is in several types of acute leukaemia, where the abnormal cells have such a strange morphology that they are described as blasts, and can be of the lymphoid or neutrophil family.

What are white cells for ?

White cells

Neutrophils

As previously indicated, white blood cells are responsible for defending us from attack by micro-organisms, and also in repair and reconstruction following tissue damage. There is little disagreement that the main function of neutrophils is to defend us from bacteria and other micro-organisms, and they do this by ingesting them, a process known as phagocytosis. Indeed, neutrophils may also be known as phagocytes. Consequently, high numbers of neutrophils are often associated with bacterial infections, but may also be found in auto-immune diseases. This is because in arthritis, the immune and inflammatory systems foolishly decide to attack the body's own tissues (such as the skin and joints) instead of bacteria. Increased levels in the absence of an infection, such as after surgery or severe exercise, may be explained as part of the body's normal response to physical stress, the so-called 'acute phase response', and such raised levels can be expected to fall back to normal as the cause of the stress subsides.

Lymphocytes

There are two major types of lymphocytes: B lymphocytes make immunoglobulins (antibodies – proteins designed to recognise, attack, and help destroy invading pathogens) whilst T lymphocytes co-operate in antibody production and also attack cells that are infected with viruses. Whilst many lymphocytes are present in the blood, they are also to be found in lymph nodes, the bone marrow, the liver and the spleen. These organs are collectively called 'lymphoid tissue'. Mildly increased numbers of lymphocytes in the blood may be expected in conditions that also cause a raised neutrophil count. However, the highest levels often encountered in health are found during attack against viral infections, such as in glandular fever. In such cases these 'activated' lymphocytes may be larger than usual, and sufficiently larger for them to be described as blasts. However, some viruses actually kill lymphocytes, so that the number in the blood will fall – HIV being such a virus.

Monocytes

Monocytes also defend us from infection by the phagocytosis of bacteria, fungi, and other pathogens, but this also occurs in tissues such as the skin, liver, and lung, where they are described as macrophages. Monocytes also co-operate with lymphocytes in making antibodies, and increased numbers can be present in chronic bacterial and protozoal infections, and in malignancy.

The last two types of normal cells are present at low levels. Eosinophils defend us against infections by large parasites, and are also active in allergy, hay fever, asthma and skin diseases. High numbers of basophils are rare but may be present in acute hypersensitivity and atopic reactions, and in some leukaemias.

Inflammation and Immunity

Inflammation and immunity

Thus neutrophils, lymphocytes and monocytes defend us from the vast majority of microbial pathogens. However, this type of defence can be viewed as having two parts. An inflammatory response often sees a large number of neutrophils being rapidly mobilised to attack a localised bacterial infection, although such a local response may escape into the blood and lead to septicaemia.

Unfortunately, these neutrophils are often a little too enthusiastic and local tissues can also be damaged or destroyed alongside the pathogens. As mentioned, lymphocytes make antibodies and attack cells that are infected with viruses, such as will be present in diseases as diverse as influenza, measles, viral hepatitis and HIV infection.

A good example of the symbiosis between the two most common types of white blood cells is where lymphocytes may make antibodies to bacteria and fungi such as yeast, which are then more palatable to the neutrophils and monocytes, thus aiding removal of these pathogens. Thus, for a full and comprehensive defence against micro-organisms, both inflammatory and immunological mechanisms are required. Infections occur when either, or both, of these processes become impaired.

Antibodies are not always good as they can take part in diseases such as rheumatoid arthritis, and often frustrate our wish to give or receive a blood transfusion (Chapter 4).

Not enough cells: leukopenia

Leukopenia

This state is often described when the WBCC falls to less than, for example, 3.7×10^9/L. However, recall that the definition of the normal range may well include some individuals with leukopenia who are entirely healthy. Nevertheless, persistently low levels are very rare in the absence of a clear explanation.

In clinical practice, virtually all cases of leukopenia are associated with the use of cytotoxic drugs such as are used in the treatment of solid cancers, leukaemia, and to aid the success of a transplant. These drugs can cause the destruction of different types of white blood cells. However, low numbers of neutrophils (i.e. neutropenia) can also be associated with supposedly benign drugs such as anti-inflammatory drugs. In such cases, the cause is therefore reasonably apparent. It follows that prophylactic antibiotic therapy is often needed in such patients. However, other drugs can cause the selective loss of lymphocytes (i.e. lymphopenia), and as such these subjects may be at risk of viral infections.

As discussed, low levels of white blood cells are also to be found in aplastic anaemia, a condition where the entire bone marrow shuts down, and so is also associated with anaemia and low numbers of platelets.

High numbers of cells: leukocytosis

Leukocytosis

As mentioned, high levels of neutrophils and lymphocytes can be found as normal responses to infections and after surgery. The reason for the former is obvious, but the latter is an example of an acute phase response – the body believes it has been attacked, so mobilises white blood cells in case it needs to defend itself from a bacterial infection

Pathological states also associated with leukocytosis include inflammatory and autoimmune diseases such as rheumatoid arthritis and systemic lupus erythematosus. However, the highest and most serious cases of leukocytosis occur in leukaemia.

Leukaemia

Leukaemia

The high white cell count in leukaemia is not due to an abnormal or persistent response to infections, but to changes in the ways in which white blood cells develop in the bone marrow. Essentially, the leukaemic cells stop their development at a certain crucial but early stage, and enter the blood not only in an immature state, but also in increased numbers. If this process develops slowly, perhaps over years, then it is said to be chronic, with survival measurable in years. These leukaemic cells are often of a more mature phenotype.

Conversely, if the increase in the white cell count is rapid, maybe over a few weeks, then the leukaemia is said to be acute. Acute leukaemias, frequently characterised by enormous numbers of immature cells (also called blasts), are also often much more aggressive than the chronic counterpart, where the increases are more modest, and survival (unless treated appropriately) can be as short as months.

If the major cell in the leukaemia is of the neutrophils lineage, the leukaemia is described as myeloid or granulocytic. When the predominant cell is a lymphocyte, then lymphocytic leukaemia is present. However, if the leukaemia is dominated by blast cells, then it may be described as lymphoblastic. Thus for the most common we have a combination of these in abbreviations:

- AML = acute myeloid leukaemia
- CGL = chronic granulocytic leukaemia
- ALL = acute lymphocytic or lymphoblastic leukaemia
- CLL = chronic lymphocytic leukaemia

Monocytic leukaemias are rare, whilst eosinophil and basophil leukaemias are very rare indeed. Thus myeloid and lymphocytic leukaemias provide by far the most work of this kind for the Haematologist.

Because the leukaemia arises in the bone marrow, and is characterised by large numbers of these abnormal cells, then the production of other cells within this tissue is also influenced. Thus anaemia and low levels of platelets (thrombocytopenia) are invariably a consequence of leukaemia, as the tumour grows and thus squeezes out other normal tissues. However, in advanced disease, the leukaemia may escape from the bone marrow and often invade lymphoid tissues of the lymph nodes, liver and spleen, making them swollen.

Treatments are aimed at reducing the tumour burden, and are generally regimes of cytotoxic drugs. More severe leukaemias demand transplantation of fresh, 'clean' bone marrow stem cells that can be obtained from a donor (i.e. allogeneic, best from an HLA-matched donor) or from the patient themselves (i.e. an autologous transplant).

Other lymphoid neoplasia

Whilst leukaemia arises in the bone marrow, other, different types of lymphoid malignancy can be present in other lymphoid tissues around the body, such as in the liver, spleen and lymph nodes.

Lymphoma

A **lymphoma** is a malignancy of (generally) B lymphocytes. Essentially, malignant but inactive lymphocytes take over the normal structure and function of the lymph node. As these bodies are often the sites of antibody production, they are no longer able to help fight infection. A principle example of this type of cancer is a Hodgkin lymphoma. Another is a Burkitt's lymphoma, but this can also be caused by a virus.

Lymphomas are often progressive: more and more lymph nodes, often in a chain, become affected and eventually the spleen, liver and bone marrow (thus possibly leading to anaemia) can become involved. Lymphoma cells are not usually seen in the blood, so a leukocytosis is infrequent. However, a lymphoma may well deteriorate in its later stages into a disease with a leukaemic picture.

Figure 4 **The natural history of leukaemia**

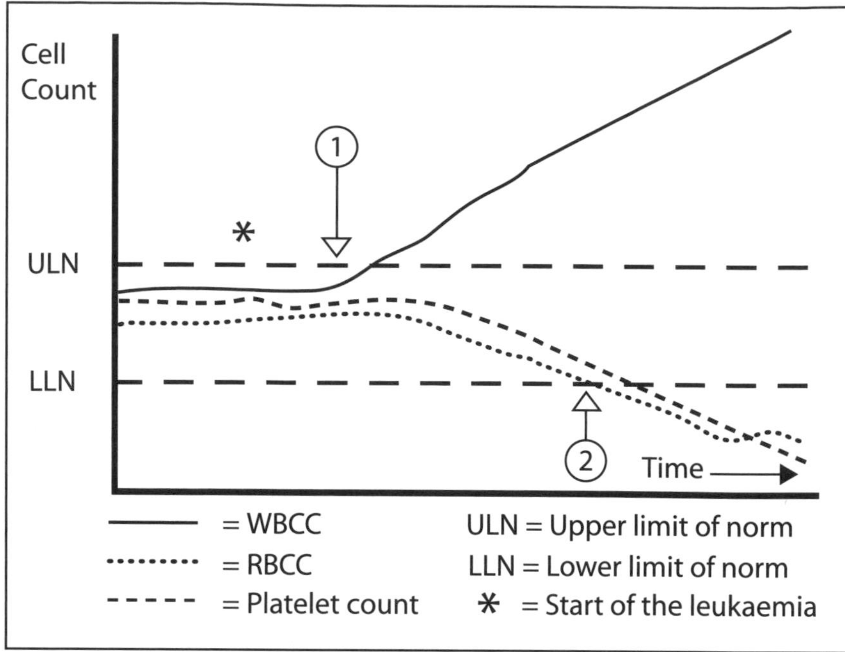

This is a representation of changes in blood cells as leukaemia progresses. The major characteristic is the slow and steady rise in WBCC, and a similar fall in RBCC and platelet count. The dotted lines are the upper and lower limits of the normal range (ULN and LLN respectively). Arrow 1 represents the start of the leukaemic process. Arrow 2 is around the time point where the red blood cell count and platelet count fall below the lower limit of normal. These are crucial points in defining a leukaemia.

We all experience minor fluctuations in blood results from day to day and week to week – hence the slight variation in the WBCC line. Indeed, levels can rise with 'normal' responses to infection, up to levels of the 'teens, say 14 or 15. However as the WBCC continues to rise to about 20 or 25 without an obvious infection (with fevers and sweating), then a malignancy becomes likely. As the WBCC progresses the patient will be suffering infections. In parallel, later in the disease, there will be falls in the RBCC and platelets (arrow two), leading eventually to the symptoms of anaemia and bruising/bleeding respectively. Eventually, these symptoms will drive the patient to seek our help, and a blood test will make the diagnosis.

Myeloma

A **myeloma** is also a tumour of the B lymphocyte that is (normally) making good antibodies to attack bacteria and viruses. However, unlike a lymphoma, this tumour is found within the bone marrow. The disease, accounting for maybe 10% of all haematological malignancies, and with a median survival of 4 years, can cause bone pain, and often so much bone is mobilised that serum calcium can rise. As the myeloma cells are making large amounts of an incorrect type of antibody, then the viscosity of the blood rises. A further consequence of this is a very high ESR. Although centred on the bone marrow, the actual tumour cells of the myeloma (plasma cells) can be found in the blood, especially in advanced disease. So a myeloma may start out (and possibly remain) centred on the bone marrow, but these myeloma cells may 'escape' (or are pushed out) into the blood. However, numbers hardly ever rise to those of a 'typical' leukaemia.

Myeloma is ultimately diagnosed by very high levels of serum immunoglobulins using a test called protein electrophoresis, often performed in the Biochemistry laboratory. In some cases, only a small part of the quite large antibody molecule is produced in excess amounts, and this can be detected in the blood or in the urine. This fraction of an entire antibody molecule is called 'Bence-Jones Protein' after its discoverer.

Websites: **www.lymphoma.org.uk** and **www.myeloma.org.uk**

Summary of white blood cells

Summary

- White blood cells defend us from infections, when raised levels of these cells (mostly neutrophils and lymphocytes) can be found in the blood.
- The most serious disease associated with inappropriately high levels is leukaemia, a condition where anaemia and low platelets are also often present.
- Other cancers of white blood cells are lymphoma and myeloma.

Case Study 2

A 22-year-old man, previously healthy, presents to his General Practitioner with an unexpected four-week history of excessive and progressive tiredness and sweating. Examination showed an inflamed throat and some lumps in his neck but no other abnormalities. The blood test result was as follows:

Haemoglobin	10.4 g/dL	**WBCC**	73.4 x 10^9/L
Platelets	117 x 10^9/L	**ESR**	33 mm/hour
Plasma viscosity	1.61 mPa	**RBCC**	4.05 x 10^{12}/L

Differential:

	Numbers (x10^9/L)	**Percentage of the WBCC**
Neutrophils	7.8	10.7
Lymphocytes	17.5	23.9
Monocytes	1.4	1.9
Eosinophils	0	0
Basophils	0	0
Blasts	46.6	63.5

As before, see page 125 for the normal ranges of these indices, find out which are abnormal, and then make your interpretation.

Interpretation

The abnormal results are low haemoglobin and platelets, with raised WBCC and ESR. The red cell count is also low. The non-appearance of eosinophils and basophils is not that surprising in view of the huge numbers of the other cells, and in this case is not clinically significant. The differential reports a low percentage of neutrophils and high numbers of blasts.

Thus with all three of the triad of leukaemia present, the initial diagnosis is not difficult. Anaemia and low platelets (thrombocytopenia) are due to the effects of the malignant leukaemia taking over the bone marrow so that the production of the other cells is reduced. A raised ESR and low red cell count support the diagnosis but add nothing new. The normal plasma viscosity also provides no new perspective. Because the onset is rapid (four week history), we suspect an acute leukaemia, and as the major cell present in lymphoid, we finally diagnose acute lymphocytic or lymphoblastic leukaemia. With such a very high white cell count, prognosis is poor.

Chapter 3

Coagulation

Key words:

Platelets
Fibrinogen
Prothrombin time (PT)
Partial thromboplastin time (PTT)
International normalised ratio (INR)

Key pathological expressions:

Thrombocytopenia
Thrombocytosis
Haemorrhage
Thrombosis
Anti-thrombotic drugs

An explanation of terms:

Platelets

Platelets: Normal range 143 to 400 x 10^9/L

These tiny bodies are fragments of a much larger cell found only in the bone marrow (the megakaryocyte), and form a clot, or thrombus, when aggregated together with the help of the blood protein fibrin. A low platelet count (possible caused by drugs [such as quinine, sulphonamides and other antibiotics], poor production, or excessive consumption) is thrombocytopenia – a raised count is thrombocytosis, and is often present in infections and some autoimmune diseases.

Fibrinogen

Fibrinogen: Normal range from 1.5 to 4 g/L

This is one of the more important blood proteins involved in clotting and is made in the liver. It is converted into fibrin by an enzyme, thrombin (itself derived from prothrombin), and is crucial in clot formation. Increased levels are found in inflammation and in smokers, decreased levels due to consumption as part of forming a clot.

Prothrombin time

Prothrombin time (PT): Normal range 11–14 seconds, and partial thromboplastin time (PTT): Normal range 24–34 seconds

The PT and PTT are laboratory measures of the ability of blood plasma to form a clot. The result provided is the time taken (in the laboratory, not in the body) for the clot to form. The difference between PT and PTT is that they measure different parts of the clotting pathway, can investigate bleeding disorders and can also be used to monitor the effects of different drugs that interfere with different parts of the coagulation system (i.e. the anticoagulants warfarin [by PT] and heparin [by PTT]). Some labs place an 'A' for activated in front of the PTT, thus APTT.

International normalised ratio

International normalised ratio (INR): Target range 2–3 or 3–4

The most widely used anticoagulant that can be given by mouth is warfarin. It works by interfering with the ability of the liver to synthesise proteins involved in clotting, so that, in the laboratory, clotting takes longer to happen. The INR is simply the ratio between the time blood takes to clot normally, compared to the (supposedly increased) time it takes to clot due to warfarin. So if a normal clotting time (PT) is 12 seconds, and on warfarin the time is 24 seconds, then the INR is 2.0. We use the INR to strike a balance between slowing down the clot-forming process, and the use of too much warfarin, which will interfere with clotting so much that a clot may never happen (a dangerous situation to be in!). Someone at a relatively low risk of thrombosis (for example, with atrial fibrillation), or with a current deep vein thrombosis (DVT) should have an INR between 2 and 3. However, those at high risk of thrombosis, for example, with a mechanical heart valve, or someone who seems to be predisposed to clots, would generally be expected to take enough warfarin to maintain an INR between 3 and 4.

What is coagulation for?

Coagulation

Clearly, to prevent excessive blood loss. A clot is composed of two elements: platelets and fibrin. Consider a small river or stream that you need to dam. One approach would be to throw a tennis net over the steam, and then float down footballs, tennis balls, basketballs etc. Eventually, the flow of water would be impeded. In this simple metaphor, the tennis net is the fibrin, and the various balls are platelets, red blood cells and white blood cells. Clearly, the tennis net by itself would not stop much water flow, and footballs by themselves would simply be washed away. They have to work together to stop water flow, as do platelets and fibrin to form a clot. The tennis balls and footballs metaphor is far from perfect, mainly as in real life the balls would not take an active part in stopping water flow. But platelets are very active cells, and take a direct part in supporting the fibrin net and making the clot more stable.

The causes, consequences and treatments of increased tendency to form a clot

Thrombosis

Since a proper word for a clot is a thrombus, then the process that concludes with the formation of a clot is thrombosis. This can occur in the arteries or in the veins.

The consequence of an arterial thrombosis that totally blocks that vessel is an infarction. This is where the tissues downstream of the clot die because they are deprived of oxygen and glucose. So if the clot lies in an artery in the heart, a (quite possibly fatal) myocardial infarction (heart attack) follows. Similarly, a clot in an artery of the brain will cause a stroke. Clots in the legs will cause critical limb ischaemia, as well as considerable pain and, possibly, the development of gangrene. These thromboses are the mainstay of the theory of atherothrombotic disease, the process that seems destined to strike at most of us in the Western World. Doubtless almost all of us are aware of the importance of the risk factors for atherosclerosis (diabetes, smoking, hypertension, hypercholesterolaemia, obesity) that all promote clot formation.

Clots in the veins are slightly different. The principle vessels burdened are of the legs (where a deep vein thrombosis [DVT] can develop) and of the vessels of the lung (where a pulmonary embolus [PE] may arise). A DVT leads to a swollen, painful leg such that walking can be difficult, if not impossible. Blockage of a crucial lung vessel by a PE will lead to breathlessness and chest pain, and can be fatal.

There are three major drugs useful for those at risk of, and needing treatment of, thrombosis:

Aspirin

Aspirin is certainly the most commonly used drug for the treatment and prevention of arterial thrombosis. It is effective, cheap, does not require refrigeration, and one dose for all can be given orally. It is now a standard treatment for all who have already had a critical cardiovascular event. It works by reducing platelet activity, so they don't get as enthusiastic about forming a clot. However, some people are intolerant or resistant to aspirin, and so need other drugs, such as clopidogrel, to suppress their platelets.

Warfarin

Vitamin K, normally obtained in our diet, is an essential requirement in our ability to synthesise key molecules involved in coagulation. So if our diet is deficient in this vitamin, we can't make the coagulation factors as efficiently and so don't form clots that well. **Warfarin** works by inhibiting this synthesis activity, so the result is the same – low levels of clotting proteins and so a long time to form a clot. This translates, in real terms, to a protection from thrombosis. .

As mentioned above, the international normalised ratio (INR) is a simple number that compares the time taken for the blood to clot whilst an individual is on warfarin, compared with the time when he or she is not on the drug. Despite its excellent efficacy, its use is plagued by risk of bleeding and by the variability of the dose between different people: some can be taking 1 mg a day whilst others take 15 mg daily to make their blood equally anticoagulated. Consequently, most patients need to attend an out-patient clinic about every 4 weeks to check that they are taking the right amount of warfarin for their particular INR. However, a serious but rare side effect of warfarin is skin necrosis, often demanding surgery. (See plates 1 and 2 opposite.)

Heparin

Heparin is a natural anticoagulant – we all have it in our blood. However, giving extra heparin will help those at risk of thrombosis, such as immediately after orthopaedic surgery. A disadvantage with this agent is that it can't be taken by mouth, so must be given by sub-cutaneous injection, or intravenously. A further problem is that it can cause dangerously low levels of platelets, and so excessive bleeding, a condition called *heparin induced thrombo-cytopenia.* If this happens, heparin is withdrawn and another anti-coagulant, such as one like hirudin (derived from the leech), can be used instead. Like warfarin, the efficacy of heparin can vary from person to person, so it must be monitored in the laboratory by the PTT test.

Recently, a safer form of heparin – **low molecular weight heparin** – has been introduced. Although it cannot be taken orally, it is safe enough to be given by subcutaneous injection, even in out-patient clinics and (for the appropriately trained patient) at home, and does not need to be monitored by the PTT test. There is also a reduced incidence of heparin-induced thrombocytopenia. There is now a form of LMWH that need be given only once a week.

Necrosis

Warfarin can cause necrosis of the skin that often needs surgical intervention

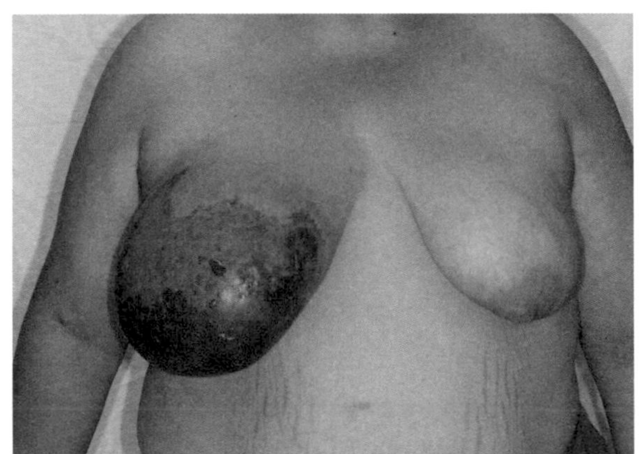

1

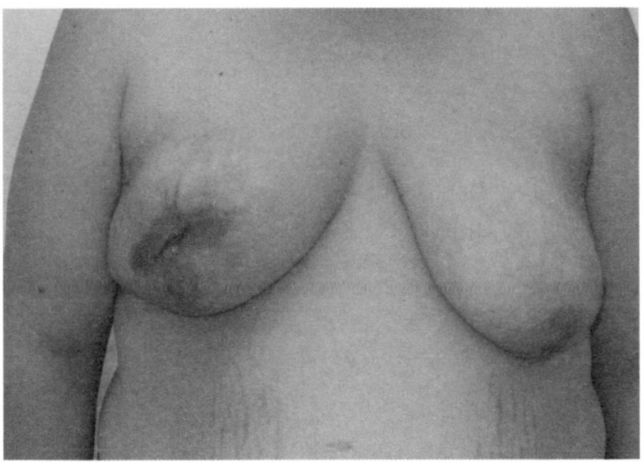

2

At the practical level, in hospital, patients coming out of surgery (and therefore at risk of thrombosis) are often started immediately on both heparin and warfarin. This double approach is needed because heparin acts almost immediately, whereas warfarin takes several days to become effective and thus protect against a clot. Once the INR has reached its target (generally 2–3), heparin may be withdrawn. Although the benefits of warfarin and heparin in terms of protection against a thrombus are clear, there is also a risk of over-anticoagulation and thus excess (possibly fatal) bleeding that must be weighed against.

Alternatively, other patients may be protected by LMWH only whilst in hospital and be discharged with their own supply so they can dose themselves at home. This self-dosing is becoming attractive as there is a long history of people with diabetes confidently and safely dosing themselves with insulin.

All these anti-thrombotic and anti-coagulant drugs have side effects, principally haemorrhage, when used in excess or in other situations. As mentioned, unfractionated heparin can cause a thrombocytopenia and warfarin a skin necrosis.

The causes, consequences and treatments of reduced ability to form a clot

Haemorrhage

Haemorrhage is the medical term for bleeding, and we have just noted that excessive anticoagulation with heparin, aspirin and warfarin can cause minor (e.g. bruising or nosebleeds) or more serious bleeding (with blood loss so severe that it may demand a blood transfusion). Fortunately, bleeding due to aspirin and heparin can often be managed by withdrawing the drug, but because the effects of warfarin are long-lasting, then the antidote is to give vitamin K orally or by injection.

The best-known coagulation gene defect is haemophilia, caused by lack of a certain crucial component of the coagulation system, Factor VIII. Without this factor, bleeding is frequent. Fortunately, the disease is rare and, although always serious, is becoming easier to treat by giving replacements of Factor VIII that are made by genetic engineering. This revolutionary technology can also provide other clotting factors, such as recombinant Factor VII, which can be used to treat a variety of bleeding disorders.

The most common inherited bleeding disorder is von Willebrand's disease, caused by lack of von Willebrand factor. Unlike haemophilia, this condition is very variable, ranging from virtually asymptomatic to life-threatening. If recombinant clotting factors are unavailable, then excessive bleeding and haemorrhage can be treated with fresh frozen plasma or cryoglobulins, which are purified and prepared from blood transfusion donations. Transfusion of purified platelets is also possible, and all these are generally from the blood bank. This is reviewed in the chapter on blood transfusion that follows.

Fibrinolysis and D-dimers

Fibrinolysis and D-dimers

Although these notes are designed to answer questions about the 'routine' full blood count, it is foolish to ignore other closely related and important topics merely because they do not yet appear on routine report forms.

Once a clot has formed, and has done its job in stemming blood loss, it must be removed by a process called fibrinolysis. The enzyme plasmin will degrade the clot into small pieces so that blood flow can be restored. Plasmin derives from an inactive precursor, plasminogen, by the activity of tissue plasminogen activator (tPA). The current treatment of a heart attack, that is presumed to follow from a clot in one of the arteries of the heart, is to give tPa (or a closely related product such as streptokinase or alteplase) to help get rid of the clot that is causing the obstruction and the associated symptoms.

A consequence of fibrinolysis is the appearance of bits of chopped-up clots in the plasma. These can be detected in the laboratory, and of these fragments, D-dimers are the most useful. Thus increased D-dimers are evidence of fibrinolysis, and so of the presence of a clot being resolved. DVT is caused by a clot in one of the veins of the leg. Thus, resolution of the DVT by the body's own repair mechanisms should be accompanied by raised levels of D-dimers. The trouble is that many conditions, including cancer, diabetes, smoking and atherosclerosis, are also accompanied by raised D-dimers, so the test is not specific for a DVT. However, around the other way, this test can be used to exclude a DVT as it is just about impossible to have normal D-dimers levels and a DVT.

Case Study 3

A 64-year old woman has elective hip-replacement surgery. She loses a bit of blood so is 'topped up' with a unit of packed red blood cells. Her recovery is good and she is maintained after her operation with analgesia and unfractionated heparin. However, she was discharged from hospital as late as day 15. What happened?

Serial post-op bloods

	Pre-op	Day 2	Day 5	Day 7	Day 9	Day 12	Day 60	Day 200
WBCC	5.9	12.1	8.5	6.6	5.5	5.8	5.5	4.0
ESR	5	15	8	6	4	5	2	4
Platelets	245	235	140	105	165	212	200	221
PT	12	10.5	15.2	17.7	12.7	12.5	31.5	12.3
PTT	30	65	70	68	69	71	28.5	29.5

WBCC = white blood cell count. ESR = erythrocyte sedimentation rate. Units for PT and PTT are seconds. The target for the PT is to give an INR of between 2 and 3. Similarly, the target for the PTT ratio is to be between 1.5 and 2.5. See page 125 for the normal ranges of these indices, Find out which are abnormal, and then make your interpretation.

Interpretation

On day two we see the expected small rise in the WBCC and ESR after surgery, with subsequent reductions on days 5 and 7, and roughly normal levels thereafter. However, the platelet count is starting to fall on day 5, is definitely low on day 7, and is improved on day 9 and thereafter. The prothrombin time (PT) is mildly prolonged on days 5 and 7, definitely on day 60, and the PTT is prolonged immediately after surgery until day 12.

The initial picture is unremarkable with a rise in PTT because of the use of unfractionated heparin, giving a PTT ratio of about 2.3. On day 5 the effects of warfarin are starting to be evident with a slightly prolonged PT (i.e. INR perhaps 1.3, aiming for 2–3). However, the big problem is the fall in the platelet count, of which the most likely cause is heparin induced thrombocytopenia. Thus the heparin would need to be withdrawn and an alternative anti-coagulant used (e.g. a hirudin, derived from the mouthparts of the leech). At the same time, warfarin (causing INR 1.5) would also be removed.

The withdrawal of heparin has a beneficial effect on the platelet count, which recovers, rising on day 9 and is normal by day 12. Day 60 sees a prolonged PT (INR 2.6) due to the re-introduction of warfarin and cessation of the drug that was used in place of heparin. By day 200 the six-month course of treatment is over and all indices are within the normal range.

Summary of coagulation

Summary

- The coagulation system exists to minimise blood loss by creating a clot (thrombus) to plug up the hole.
- The clot is composed of platelets in a mesh of fibrin that may also include red blood cells.
- Excessive and inappropriate clotting can lead to possibly fatal disease, and can be retarded by drugs such as aspirin, warfarin and heparin.
- Fibrinolysis is the dissolution of the clot, and leads to raised D-dimers, molecules that can be used to exclude a DVT.

Figure 5

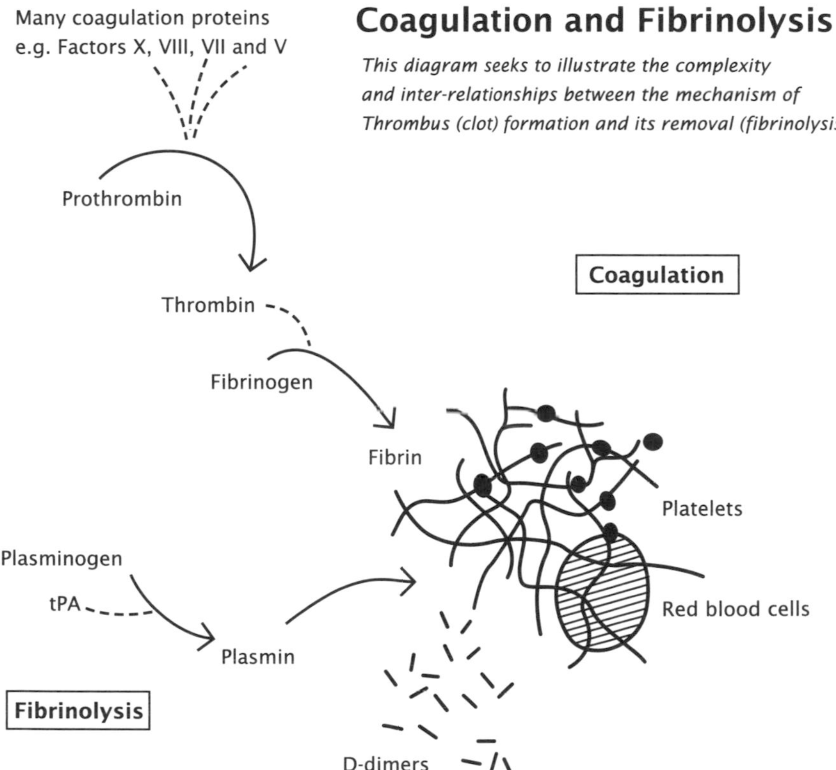

Chapter 4

Blood Transfusion

Key words:

ABO blood groups
Antibodies
Cross-match
Group and Save
Rhesus blood group

Key pathological expressions:

Anaemia
Sickle cell disease
Transfusion reaction

An explanation of terms:

Blood transfusion

This short section summarises key aspects of blood transfusion. Clearly, this is not so much a blood test, but a form of therapy. But equally clearly it belongs within the realm of haematology, and so is deserving of inclusion.

The objective of blood transfusion has changed markedly over the years, from being an instrument to keep up the haemoglobin level, to a therapy to save lives. Additional changes have been the realisation that this is far from a simple and trouble-free treatment but one that can damage, possibly permanently, the health of the recipient.

A further development has been the move from transfusing 'whole' blood, which therefore included plasma (with all its proteins and antibodies), white blood cells and platelets, to transfusing only specific components, usually just the red blood cells. The latter, called 'packed cells', is not only more efficient, but also, without the white blood cells and (possibly damaging) plasma antibodies, produces fewer adverse reactions. Furthermore, the 'leftover' plasma from a blood donation can provide other useful blood products (such as clotting proteins) although these can also be produced by genetic engineering.

Blood groups

Blood Groups

The ABO and rhesus (Rh) blood group systems consist of two parts; firstly molecules (antigens) that are present at the surface of the cell and are a type of identification, related in theory to the HLA system, but are far simpler, and secondly a series of antibodies that recognise these molecules.

ABO system

The ABO system

Antigens A and B are structures with different 'sugars' at the end that can be present on the surface of red blood cells. If you have only the blood group A structure on your red blood cells, you are blood group A. Similarly, if you have only group B molecules on your red cells then you are group B. People with both A and B molecules on their red blood cells are group AB, and if you have neither of these structures on your red cells, you are group O.

We also have antibodies in our plasma that recognise blood group structures A and B, but in the healthy individual, these are the reverse of your blood group. So if you are group A, you will have antibodies that will recognise group B (i.e. Anti-B). Likewise, group B people have antibodies that recognise group A (i.e. Anti-A). Group AB people have no antibodies, but group O people have both anti-A and anti-B antibodies in their plasma.

This is summarised in Table 3.

ABO Blood Group

Table 3
Determinants of ABO Blood Group

Blood Group	Antigen structures on the red blood cell surface	Antibodies in the plasma
A	A	Anti-B
B	B	Anti-A
AB	A and B	No antibodies present
O	No antigens present	Both anti-A and anti-B are present

The Rhesus system

Rhesus system

The Rh system is very much more complicated, being composed of perhaps 48 recognised antigens, although on a day to day basis, only five different structures on the surface of the blood cell are commonly dealt with in the blood bank. A full explanation of this is beyond the scope of this simple book. However, in practice, we tend to focus on the molecule known as D (i.e. Rh D), as it is this structure and the antibodies that it can generate that can give rise to haemolytic disease of the newborn if not correctly treated. Other members of the Rhesus family of antigens are C, c̄, E and ē.

The main distinction between the ABO and Rh systems is that in the normal person, there are ALWAYS antibodies to absent antigens. This makes ABO incompatible transfusions potentially fatal.

Why order a blood transfusion?

As mentioned, in the past this was simply because the attending physician considered it a good thing to do, that it would probably do the patient some good. This would, of course, be fine but for a number of problems. To name but a few:

- In practice, whilst the ABO/Rh systems are the most important, there are a host of other blood group antigens (with names such as Duffy and Kell) that can be a problem. The more transfused a person becomes, then the greater the likelihood that antibodies to these minor groups can build up to be a real clinical and laboratory issue.

- We are programmed to collect and save iron in stores all over the body. People who are hyper-transfused often have problems in various organs as the build up of this iron can cause damage to the tissues.

- Transfused blood can contain pathogenic organisms such as viruses (hepatitis B and C, HIV), although, gladly, due to screening, this is becoming less of a problem.

Therefore, not simply because of the above, the present view is that blood transfusion should be reserved only for those in danger of losing their life, or who will show a measurable improvement not achievable by other means, and the earlier case report of a woman with sickle cell disease underlines this point. It follows that the requirement for a transfusion can only be made clinically, not in the laboratory. However, much experience is available within the blood bank and advice should be sought if cases fall outside established practice or guidelines.

Cross-match

Cross-match

So assuming your patient needs (or will/may be in need of) a blood transfusion, what blood tests are required? It is important to match the blood group of the person needing the transfusion (the recipient) with the group of the blood that is to be transfused. This process is called a cross-match, and is done in the blood bank on a sample of the patient/recipients' EDTA or clotted blood. If in doubt about which blood tube to use, ring the Laboratory.

The essential steps are:

(a) the patient must be ABO and Rh (D) typed
(b) there must be screening for clinically significant antibodies (this is more important than the cross-match)
(c) the actual cross-match is where patient plasma or serum is tested against potential donors.

In practice, your colleagues in the blood bank will mix blood from the patient (recipient) with a series of stored bloods (often 5 or 6) from different donors, to see if there are any matches. A good match is where the red blood cells are unaltered by this mixing, and therefore should not react when in the patient. However, blood that does not match will aggregate, forming small clots, indicating an incompatibility. This is inevitably because the antigens on the red blood cells and the antibodies in the serum recognise each other, and react together, causing blood to clump.

An example of this would be mixing blood from someone of blood group A with that of someone of blood group B. The group

A person has group A molecules on their red cells but also antibodies against B in the plasma (i.e. Anti-B). The group B person has the reverse – group B molecules on their red cells and anti-A antibodies in their plasma. So, when mixed, the group A red cells will be recognised by the anti-A antibodies, and so will react together. Similarly, the group B red blood cells will be recognised by the anti-B, and will also react. Recall from the section on antibodies in the white blood cells chapter that the purpose of antibodies is often to attack and destroy anything they react with. Hence the danger.

The same principle of incompatibility also occurs in other systems, such as antibodies to a Rh antigen or to a Kell antigen being reactive with (respectively) specific anti-Rh or anti-Kell antibodies.

So if any of this incompatible donor blood were to be transfused into the patient/recipient, the clumping or destruction of red blood cells observed in the laboratory would also happen in the recipient, causing an adverse transfusion reaction. This is often heralded by symptoms such as fevers, chills, shaking, shortness of breath, headache, pain etc. This can be followed by more severe clinical situations (such as collapse, hypotension, renal failure and pulmonary oedema) that could be fatal. Consequently, many hospitals have a policy of at least two members of staff checking the blood they are about to transfuse into one of their patients. This approach has proven to reduce mistake and serious hazards of transfusion. Many wards and hospitals have their own formal policy, and professional bodies (e.g. Royal College of Nursing) generally offer guidelines.

Group and Save

Group and Save

The request 'Group and Save' is simply an extension of the request for a cross-match. This instruction is to find out the patient's blood group (Group), as discussed above, but then keep the blood handy (Save, generally in a refrigerator) as it is likely to be needed in a cross-match in the near future. A Group and Save is often requested of patients about to undergo surgery in the next few days or weeks, so that the laboratory has a head start in trying to match some stored blood for the patient.

Blood Products

Blood products

As discussed in Chapter 3, the Blood Bank can provide not only red blood cells, but also platelets and coagulation proteins such as fibrinogen, factor VIII, factor VII, fresh frozen plasma (FFP) and cryoprecipitate. These will be needed by people at risk of haemorrhage, or with actual haemorrhagic blood loss, but who do not need red blood cells, such as those with haemophilia and severe von Willebrand's disease. As fragments of cells, platelets will also need to be checked for blood group compatibility. Albumin (generally as a 20% preparation) is also available for people with low levels or who have had heavy burns (although only regional centres will deal with these risky patients) or ascites.

All hospitals will deal with haemorrhage due to prolonged prothrombin time, partial thromboplastin time, decreased fibrinogen, over-anticogulation with warfarin or heparin, trauma, surgery, disseminated intravascular coagulation, etc.

Summary of Blood Transfusion

Summary

- This therapy is generally reserved for urgent and life-threatening clinical situations such as blood loss. It is now rarely seen as a temporary 'cure' for anaemia where an alternative such as iron may be preferable.
- Blood groups are A, B, AB and O, but Rhesus D is also important
- Requests are usually to 'group and save', and to 'cross-match'
- The blood bank also provides platelets, albumin and coagulation factors
- You also have access to highly specialised services in investigating reactions and providing ultra-specialist products, e.g. HLA matched platelets, stem cells etc.

Chapter 5

Haematology Case Reports

As for the previous case studies, see page 125 for the normal ranges of these indices, find out which of them are abnormal, and then make your interpretation. Answers start on page 49.

Case report 1

A 35-year-old man presents with a six-week history of intermittent general lethargy with fevers, generalised aches and pains, loose stools and abdominal discomfort. He had recently returned from a prolonged period 'backpacking' in the tropics. Both the liver and spleen were slightly enlarged.

Haemoglobin	14.5 g/dL	**RBCC**	4.8 x 10^{12}/L
WBCC	16.6 x 10^9/L	**Platelets**	242 x 10^9/L
ESR	15 mm/hour	**MCV**	88.6 fL

		Absolute	**% of the WBCC**
Differential:	Neutrophils	13.5 x 10^9/L	81.3
	Lymphocytes	1.2	7.2
	Monocytes	0.4	2.4
	Eosinophils	1.5	9.0
	Basophils	0.1	< 1
	Blasts	0.1	< 1

Case report 2

A 65-year-old man gave his family doctor a one-year history of chronic ill health characterised by infections requiring antibiotics and recurrent bouts of left middle abdominal aching pain. Three days before presentation, he had noticed skin bruises, and on the day of visiting his doctor, he had, for the first time, a spontaneous nosebleed. On examination, there was a mild splenomegaly. Bloods were taken:

Haemoglobin	9.2 g/dL	**WBCC**	36 x 10^9/L
RBCC	4.1 x 10^{12}/L	**Platelets**	85 x 10^9/L
PT	13 seconds	**PTT**	29 seconds

		Absolute	**% of the WBCC**
Differential:	Neutrophils	1.1 x 10^9/L	3.0
	Lymphocytes	7.3	20.2
	Monocytes	0.5	1.8
	Eosinophils	none	0
	Basophils	none	0
	Blasts	27.1	75.0

Case report 3

A 20-year-old student presents with a week's onset of influenza-like symptoms, with general malaise, pyrexia, an intermittent skin rash, sore throat (but no lumps) and an unspecified arthralgia but no swollen joints. A recent urinary tract infection had previously responded to oral antibiotics. As the present symptoms seemed to be more severe and persistent than general 'flu, a blood test was performed:

Haemoglobin	13.8 g/dL	**Platelets**	350 x 10^9/L
WBCC	18 x 10^9/L	**RBCC**	5.0 x 10^{12}/L
Hct	48 %	**ESR**	23 mm/hour
Fibrinogen	2.5 mg/dL	**Plasma viscosity**	1.59 mPa

		Absolute	**% of the WBCC**
Differential:	Neutrophils	4.3 x 10^9/L	23.9
	Lymphocytes	9.8	54.4
	Monocytes	1.5	8.3
	Eosinophils	0.3	1.7
	Basophils	0.1	0.6
	Blasts	2.0	11.1

(n.b. is the sex of the student relevant to this report?)

Case report 4

An 8-year-old girl is noted to bleed excessively after an operation to remove her tonsils. Neither she, nor her family, have ever had any problems with excessive bleeding, and her mother did not recall any bleeds after the usual childhood traumas. Her mother and elder sister (age 17) report normal menstrual bleeding, and her mother did not report excessive bleeding after childbirth. After having recovered from her surgery several weeks later, her blood results were as follows.

Haemoglobin	13.2 g/dL	**WBCC**	4.3 x 10^9/L
Platelets	295 x 10^9/L	**RBCC**	4.5 x 10^{12}/L
MCV	84 fL	**MCHC**	32.3 pg/dL
MCH	27.1 pg	**Hct**	37.8 %
PTT	54 seconds	**PT**	12 seconds
Fibrinogen	2.8 mg/dL	**ESR**	3 mm/hour

Case report 5

A 60-year-old man, slightly overweight, with a long-standing mechanical prosthetic aortic valve replacement complained of breathlessness, being tired, occasional 'dark urine' and ankle swelling whilst at a routine visit to the anti-coagulant clinic. The full blood count was:

Haemoglobin	11.2 g/dL	**WBCC**	9.8 x 10^9/L
Platelets	336 x 10^9/L	**RBCC**	4.5 x 10^{12}/L
MCV	90 fL	**MCHC**	25.2 pg/dL
MCH	22.6 pg	**Hct**	40.5 %
PTT	35 seconds	**PT**	40 seconds
Fibrinogen	3.0 mg/dL	**ESR**	15 mm/hour

The blood film shows red blood cell fragments.

Case report 6

A 50-year-old woman with long-term Crohn's disease, on various treatments and with an abdominal surgical history, had the following test results following a routine GP visit where she complained of some lethargy, fevers and diarrhoea.

Haemoglobin	10.5 g/dL	**RBCC**	4.1 x 10^{12}/L
WBCC	9.1 x 10^9/L	**Platelets**	350 x 10^9/L
MCV	72 fL	**Hct**	29.5 %
MCHC	35.9 g/dL	**MCH**	25.6 pg
ESR	26 mm/hour	**Fibrinogen**	4.5 mg/dL

The low haemoglobin was followed up with an assessment of iron status:

Serum iron 5.8 μmol/L (normal range 10–31 μmol/L)

Case report 7

A 75-year-old woman, living alone and with a body mass index of 18.5, complains of slowly developing fatigue so that she has difficulty getting out. On examination, there is a swollen and painful tongue, and she complains of occasional 'tingling' of her fingertips, and numbness in her toes. Routine bloods were:

Haemoglobin	9.6 g/dL	**WBCC**	5.5 x 10^9/L
Platelets	198 x 10^9/L	**MCV**	108 fL
MCHC	21.3 pg/dL	**MCH**	26.5 pg
ESR	19 mm/hour	**Hct**	45 %

In view of her signs, symptoms and history, additional bloods were requested:

Serum vitamin B_{12} 98 pg/mL (normal range 145–914 pg/mL)

Serum iron 12.8 μmol/L (normal range 10–31 μmol/L)

Case report 8

A 55-year-old man complains to his GP of frequent headaches. He smokes 20 cigarettes a day and drinks 20 pints of beer a week. On examination he is overweight, with a red face and thread veins, and systolic/diastolic blood pressure of 160/100 mmHg. His breathing is very shallow. Otherwise, there is nothing abnormal detected. Bloods were:

Haemoglobin	18.5 g/dL	**Hct**	56 %
MCHC	33.0 g/dL	**MCV**	81 fL
MCH	26.8 pg		
RBCC	6.9 x 10^{12}/L	**WBCC**	9.2 x 10^9/L
Platelets	374 x 10^9/L	**Fibrinogen**	4.5 g/L

Case report 9

The case is a 63-year-old man who is obese. He reports being a non-smoker but a consumer of 2 pints of beer on a Saturday night, and complains of lethargy. However, he is particularly unhelpful in responding to other questions, such as any fevers or sweating, answering in monosyllables and short sentences, claiming to 'all right'.

Haemoglobin	13.4 g/L	**WBCC**	23.7 x 10^9/L
Platelets	135 x 10^9/L	**MCV**	102 fL
ESR	15 mm/hour	**Hct**	48 %

Differential:		**Absolute**	**% of the WBCC**
	Neutrophils	17.8 x 10^9/L	75.1
	Lymphocytes	1.3	5.5
	Monocytes	4.1	17.3
	Eosinophils	0.4	1.7
	Basophils	0.1	0.4

Other tests:

Serum Vitamin B_{12} 700 pg/mL (normal range 145–914 pg/mL)

Serum iron 14.1 µmol/L (normal range 10–31 µmol/L)

Case report 10

A 79-year-old woman is admitted with respiratory distress, possibly pneumonia. Found to be a little dehydrated, practitioners are concerned about possible progression to actual pneumonia as haemophilus influenzae is isolated. Thus, high dose antibiotics are started. However, after 48 hours she develops a rash and in the following 24 hours has some nosebleeds. Bloods were ...

Haemoglobin	11.2 g/dL	**WBCC**	10.1×10^9/L
Platelets	88×10^9/L	**RBCC**	4.2×10^{12}/L
MCH	26.7 pg	**Hct**	37.9%
MCV	90.2 fL	**MCHC**	29.6 g/dL
PTT	35 seconds	**PT**	12 seconds
Fibrinogen	3.0 mg/dL	**ESR**	18 mm/hour

Solutions to Haematology Case Reports

Solutions

Case report 1

Abnormal results are raised WBCC and ESR, with increased numbers of neutrophils and eosinophils. The most likely explanation is a bacterial or parasitic infection, possibly in the intestines, that may be confirmed by finding parasites and/or their eggs in faeces. If there were raised lymphocytes, we might have thought of a viral infection, but the subject claims good vaccinations, generally against viruses. Malaria could be present, and is not always associated with an anaemia. Amoebic dysentery a possibility?

Case report 2

Major features are the low haemoglobin, platelets and RBCC with a high WBCC. The differential shows high numbers (but low percentage) of lymphocytes, and high numbers and percentage of blast cells. Thus the preliminary diagnosis is leukaemia, supported by the symptoms, pointing to a chronic presentation. Nosebleeds often follow a platelet count less than 100. There is also a reduction in numbers and percentage of neutrophils, probably following the overall suppression of normal bone marrow by the leukaemic cells.

Case report 3

The only abnormal findings are raised WBCC, due mostly increased lymphocytes, and the raised ESR, both consistent with a viral infection. The high numbers of blasts are not necessarily a concern as they may be activated lymphocytes involved in anti-viral work. There is no anaemia or low platelets, so this is not leukaemia. Plasma viscosity is normal and adds nothing. A likely preliminary diagnosis is glandular fever, also known as infectious mononucleosis, confirmable with the monospot or Paul Bunel test.

The sex is irrelevant for the haemoglobin, as it is above the bottom of the normal range for both men and women. However, the haematocrit is slightly above the normal range for women, but is within the normal range for men. Thus, we hope the case is a young man.

Case report 4

There are no problems with this girl's red blood cells, ESR, white blood cells or platelets. Her PTT is prolonged but her PT and fibrinogen levels are acceptable. This points to a specific defect, probably a missing coagulation factor, in the 'top' part of the coagulation cascade, before the steps that lead to the generation of thrombin from prothrombin (Figure 5). It is virtually impossible for females to have haemophilia, but they may have a closely related condition. However, additional tests will be necessary to find the exact deficiency, that may well be von Willebrand's disease, the most common genetic coagulation disorder. Other possibilities include defects in clotting factors XII, XI, IX, X and V. Platelet function tests may also be needed.

Case report 5

This case has a mild anaemia, raised ESR, prolonged prothrombin time but normal PTT. Red blood cell fragments suggest some physical damage, pointing to a normocytic (red cells are of normal size – see the MCV) and haemolytic anaemia. The prolonged PT translates to an INR of 3.5, which is appropriate for prophylaxis against the high risk of thrombosis in view of a mechanical heart valve, which, in turn, we presume requires attention. This would also account for his symptoms, although these may arise from other problems.

Case report 6

Abnormal findings are low haemoglobin, low MCV, MCH and MCHC and iron. There is raised ESR and fibrinogen. The patient has an inflammatory disorder that accounts for the raised ESR, but the anaemia can also contribute to this abnormality. On the other hand, we may expect the subject to be on some anti-inflammatory drugs, and the white cell count is on the high side of normal. The low MCV and poor iron status point to an iron-deficient microcytic anaemia. This may be due to poor diet but is as likely to be due to malabsorption as the patient has bowel problems and a history of abdominal surgery that may have been removal of some sections of the intestines important in the absorption of iron. Fever and diarrhoea point to a flare up in the disease (i.e. active disease), and this also accounts for the increased fibrinogen.

Case report 7

We find low haemoglobin, and MCHC but raised MCV. There is also a raised ESR with low vitamin B_{12}. Iron studies are normal, so she is not iron deficient. The key result in the raised MCV (that also accounts for the low MCHC) and therefore macrocytic anaemia. The symptoms are also supportive. Low B_{12} may be due to poor diet (note the low body mass index) or malabsorption, so that additional tests are required. The incidence of subnormal vitamin B_{12} in elderly persons is surprisingly common, ranging from 3.0 to 4.5%, depending on the diagnostic criteria used. The expression *pernicious anaemia* is reserved for the condition that follows autoimmune gastritis, and needs to be proven by additional tests. The anaemia may also account for the raised ESR, although there may be occult reasons for this (e.g. cancer or inflammation, although the white cell count is normal).

Case report 8

Abnormal findings are raised haemoglobin, red blood cell count and haematocrit, and also fibrinogen. We look now to the clinical history for clues to aetiology, and find a rather unhealthy picture with hypertension, heavy smoking and drinking. The increases in the red cell indices are therefore likely to be due to a reaction to a (smoking-induced) hypoxia, hence reactive polycythaemia. This is because tobacco smoke contains carbon monoxide, which binds irreversibily to haemoglobin, and prevents it from binding and thus carrying oxygen. Consequently, the red cell is effectively dead and is therefore a burden.

We may also predict high viscosity that, if present, will place additional stress on the heart so that left ventricular hypertrophy may develop, especially with hypertension. Raised fibrinogen could be due to smoking, and as smokers often have a mild inflammatory response, this could cause the high-ish WBCC. Lifestyle changes are required if the risk of a stroke is to be reduced.

Case report 9

Although the haemoglobin is only just within the normal range, there is a raised WBCC and ESR with platelets only just outside the normal range. There is also a macrocytosis. Most of the raised WBCC can be accounted for by neutrophils and, unusually, monocytes. The raised WBCC implies an infection, and the neutrophil leukocytosis implies a bacterial infection. This may also be supported by the slightly abnormal ESR. However, the subject denies the fever that we would have to expect with an infection generating a white cell count of this magnitude. Interpretation is therefore difficult.

Certainly, repeat bloods would be a good idea to see if the borderline low haemoglobin and platelet counts are correct. The other explanation may be the early stages of a leukaemia. If so, it seems unusual as there are both increased neutrophils and increased monocytes, although this is possible. If we do suspect a leukaemia then more complex tests will be required.

Raised MCV is curious but in the light of normal B_{12} may be due to excessive alcohol consumption. Recall that not everything that the subject says will be the truth, the whole truth and nothing but the truth! What does he drink on the other six nights?

Case report 10

The abnormal results are thrombocytopenia (platelets less than 140), with a raised ESR. The low haemoglobin and other red cell indices are suggestive of anaemia, but are not clinically crucial at present. The high-ish WBCC is barely within the normal range and this potential leukocytosis is in keeping with an infection. Most of the laboratory picture is therefore unsurprising, with the exception of the low platelets which fit in with the nose bleeds. We could be looking at a drug-induced thrombocytopenia due to the high doses of antibiotics, and the skin rash could also be a side effect. Some antibiotics, such as cefaclor, may also cause a haemolytic anaemia although one should not yet leap to conclusions in this case as the haemoglobin is only a little outside the normal range. Fortunately, such side effects are generally reversible upon withdrawal of the drug, although other antibiotics may produce the same result.

Part 2

Biochemistry

Biochemistry:
Objectives and Scope

Objectives and scope

There are many similarities between haematology and biochemistry. Indeed, the two are often described together as 'blood science'. There are also numerous instances where the pathophysiology of one spills over to influence the other – and renal disease is an excellent example of this as we shall see.

As for haematology, it is taken as understood that all blood tubes and forms must be fully labelled by those taking the blood in order to minimise the risk of (possible fatal) error. Indeed, the laboratory will be within its right to decline to test a particular sample that is incorrectly or inadequately labelled.

The major difference between these two sciences is that almost all biochemistry is done on serum obtained from clotted blood, although blood glucose is the prime example of a biochemistry test done on blood that has to be anti-coagulated. Thus testing can only be performed on blood that is collected in the correct tube. Failure to do so will, at best, result in a polite phone call from the lab explaining the problem and its remedy. At worse, a report will be returned a day or so later with a comment such as 'inappropriate blood sample received, please repeat'. Fortunately, many blood tubes have different coloured tops to help this process and minimise errors. Therefore, again, if in doubt, PHONE

Again, as for haematology, a note on units. Few of us with an interest in lipids will disagree that a total cholesterol result of 8.5 is undesirable, even though the correct terms are 8.5 mmol/L. This, however, will certainly be a problem to those (such as Americans) reporting cholesterol in different units of mg/dL. For example, their result would be 325! It matters not so much that the correct unit of, shall we say, serum calcium is given, for example, as 4.5 mmol/L, or in shorthand simply as 4.5, but it does matter that this particular result is very serious and demands immediate attention.

The objectives of the Biochemistry section follow in Table 4 overleaf.

Figure 6 Biochemistry Report Form

CLINICAL CHEMISTRY City Hospital NHS Trust Birmingham B18 7QH

Surname	BLANN	Address	Unit No.	ASCOT CLINIC ASCOT STUDY
Forename	Andrew		Not Given	
D.O.B.	11.08.54		NHS No. *	

Lab No. C.05.0230313.C

Results:

Test	Result	Units	Range
Urea	4.3	mmol/L	(3.0-8.3)
Sodium	144	mmol/L	(133-148)
Potassium	4.1	mmol/L	(3.3-5.6)
Creatinine	89	umol/L	(44-133)
Albumin	44	g/L	(35-50)
Bilirubin	4	umol/L	(<21)
Alk Phosphatase	57	iu/L	(20-130)
Alanine AT	22	iu/L	(<41)
Calcium	2.28	mmol/L	(2.20-2.60)
Free T4	16	pmol/L	(10-24)
T.S.H.	1.72	miu/L	(0.40-5.50)
PTH	55	pg/mL	(10-65)
Cholesterol	4.2	mmol/L	(2.5-5.0)
Triglycarides	0.8	mmol/L	(<2.3)
HDL-Cholesterol	1.4	mmol/L	(>1.0)

LIP2. Triglyceride ref range is for fasting patients only
PTH2. Please note new reference range for PTH wef 26.11.2003

RANDOM SAMPLE

Tests	Check Clinician	
CA, CRE, FT4N, HDL1, LFT2, LIP2, TSH, UE		Date received 12.11.05 Date reported 12.11.05

As for the haematology, this form, reporting the author's blood, was produced by the author's hospital laboratory. Once more the report offers (from left to right) a column of words and abbreviations (particular tests), a column of numbers (the result), another column of numbers and letters (units), and yet another column of numbers (the normal or target range).

Again, the main objective of this section of the book is to explain to you what all this means.

Table 4
Learning Objectives – Biochemistry

Learning objectives – biochemistry

Having completed these notes in a satisfactory manner, the reader will:

1. Appreciate that almost all biochemistry tests need to be done on serum. The principle exception is glucose.

2. Recognise the major areas of interest, i.e.
   - Fluid and electrolytes balance
   - Sodium and potassium
   - The kidney
   - Liver function tests and plasma proteins
   - Atherosclerosis and its risk factors (e.g. diabetes)
   - Calcium
   - Thyroid function

3. Describe major clinical problems associated with each of these areas, e.g., respectively
   - Dehydration
   - Renal and liver failure
   - Diabetic coma

4. Interpret simple biochemistry results, e.g.
   - A urea of 21.4 with a creatinine of 145
   - A bilirubin of 7 with an alkaline phosphatase of 890
   - A calcium of 1.9 with an albumin of 32

5. Understand the basic purpose of the Biochemistry Laboratory.

Chapter 6

Water, urea and electrolytes

Key words:

	Normal/reference range
Sodium	133–144 mmol/L
Potassium	3.4–5.1 mmol/L

Key pathological expressions:

Hypernatraemia
Hyponatraemia
Hyperkalaemia
Hypokalaemia
Dehydration

An explanation of terms:

Urea and electrolytes

Urea and electrolytes (U&E) are undoubtedly the most commonly requested biochemistry tests. Urea is the major excretory product of our biochemical metabolism, whilst creatinine is a more specialised product of the breakdown of proteins. An explanation of the role of urea and creatinine is best left for the section on renal disease that follows.

Electrolytes are charged atoms (ions) or molecules that are involved in the passage of electricity, and are often written with a small plus or minus, like Na+ and Cl-, indicating their electrical charge, although, in practice, charge is often ignored. Sodium (Na), hydrogen (H) and potassium (K) are most commonly requested whilst others, such as Cl (chloride) and HCO_3 (bicarbonate) are less frequently requested, although the latter can be important, especially in acidosis. The anion gap is (effectively) the difference between Na plus K versus Cl plus bicarbonate. It can also be argued that calcium (Ca) is an electrolyte, but it belongs in a section of its own. However, before we embark on a discussion of U&Es, we must consider water.

Water

Water

A curious place to begin, you may think, but water is fundamental to all blood tests, as the concentration [C] of any substance is given by the mass (amount) [M] of that substance divided by the volume [V] of the fluid it is dissolved in (i.e. water in blood).

$$C = \frac{M_{in} - M_{out}}{V_{in} - V_{out}}$$

In the clinical setting, however, the total mass and total volume of fluids are the difference between in (eating and drinking – M_{in} and V_{in}) and out (excreting – M_{out} and V_{out}). This means that the concentration of something is a balance and will be higher if there is more of it in a fixed volume, or if there is the same amount of it in a smaller volume. Thus biochemists often consider the state of hydration or dehydration of their patients. As we shall see, the amount of water in the blood is regulated by the kidney. Therefore problems with this organ can lead to water retention (and thus, possibly, oedema), or excess water loss (V_{out}) as too much urine is made (diuresis: leading to dehydration). Water loss as excess urine is clear, but not so easy to account for is water loss via sweat, through the lungs (especially on hot days), and in faeces (especially in diarrhoea). These small and separate (by themselves) losses of water can add up to be considerable.

Sodium

Sodium: Normal range 133–148 mmol/L

This is the primary electrolyte in the blood, as there is more of it than any other. Indeed, as such it is the major contributor to the total mass of different ions in the blood (the osmolality). Faced with increases or decreases, we need to consider the equation concentration = mass/volume, so that one good reason to have changes in serum sodium is that the diet is abnormally rich or low in this salt. Another reason is that the amount of water in the blood has increased or fallen. Since the kidney regulates both these aspects, changes in sodium may indicate problems with this organ.

Thus **hypernatraemia**, (i.e. serum sodium > 148 mmol/L) may be due to a salt rich diet (e.g. high M_{in}) and/or a degree of dehydration – the classical clinical sign of which is loss of elasticity of the skin (the pinch test – although unreliable in the elderly). However, the most common reason is water loss, possibly due to insufficient intake in drinking (i.e. low V_{in}), excess loss in urine, or losses in sweat and diarrhoea (i.e. high V_{out}). Clinically, the simplest treatment is to replace fluid orally, if possible. If this is not possible (maybe because the patient is in a coma) then water can be infused as part of a dextrose drip.

Similarly, **hyponatraemia**, (i.e. serum sodium < 133 mmol/L) may be due to retention of water (low V_{out}) and/or excessive loss of sodium (high M_{out}). For this most common in-hospital electrolyte disturbance (15% of patients), very rare causes include insufficient sodium in the diet, and very high levels of proteins or lipids in the blood. A recognised sign of this fluid retention is oedema, although this may not always be present. Oedema is also associated with heart failure and hypoalbuminaemia. In some cases, water retention can be treated with thiazide drugs, but this can be dangerous if the kidneys are not adequately functioning.

Potassium

Potassium: Normal range 3.3 – 5.6 mmol/L

Many aspects of potassium regulation are similar to sodium (such as intake and outlet), but with a number of crucial differences. The first is that the majority of our potassium is within cells, not in the plasma – the reverse of sodium. A second is the relationship between potassium and hydrogen ions: as hydrogen ions increase (as in acidosis) then potassium is displaced from the cell and enters the plasma. The reverse is true in alkalosis. Overall, (unlike sodium) potassium does not vary a great deal in response to large changes in water balance.

Hyperkalaemia (serum potassium >5.6mmol/L) may be due to renal problems (e.g. failure to excrete sufficient potassium), acidosis, or release from damaged cells (e.g. destruction of red bloods cells or tumour cells [? by chemotherapy], or crush injuries). However, whatever the reason, it may be serious as high levels (for example, >7 mmol/L) can contribute to cardiac arrest because of interference with nerves. Therefore high potassium is the most common and most serious electrolyte emergency, and treatment includes insulin and glucose to get potassium into cells. Other treatments include calcium gluconate, resonium A and dialysis.

Causes of **hypokalaemia** (serum potassium <3.3 mmol/L) include the reverse of the above, e.g. alkalosis, in addition to loss in diarrhoea and vomiting, from the kidney, or inappropriate use of corticosteroids or thiazide drugs. In the case of the latter, a reactive alkalosis may result. Treatment focuses on replacement, such as oral salts, or a potassium-rich drip supplement.

Intravenous (IV) fluids

Intravenous (IV) fluids

It follows from much of the above that loss of fluid balance is important, and can be restored by IV fluids, usually in 500 ml or 1 litre bags. Fluids may also be given to replace losses that can be predicted. Water cannot be given by itself as it will destroy red blood cells, so must be given as 5% dextrose. It will enter the blood and also move into the tissues and cells. Saline (0.9% NaCl) rehydrates plasma and lymph, but not cells, whilst plasma expanders replace fluid deficits in the blood alone. Most clinical situations can be managed with these three fluids, plus 1.26% bicarbonate (to treat acidosis) and concentrated supplements (such as potassium). However, misuse of IV fluids can, of course, cause the reverse of what is being treated, so that monitoring is crucial

Laboratory monitoring is by frequent measurement of serum electrolytes, but clinical assessment (such as pulse, blood pressure, body weight) can also be important. Measurement of fluids taken orally (by drinking) and the volume of urine produced is important, but these will not always add up to 100% due to 'insensible' losses that are not easy to calculate (from sweat, lungs, and in faeces). Also, if someone is vomiting, this will also compound a possible state of dehydration.

Summary of Water, Urea and Electrolytes

Summary

- Overall, U&Es are often used to monitor renal function
- Consider the equation concentration = mass/volume of water
- Hypernatraemia may be due to decreased water intake, increased sodium intake, or decreased sodium intake with greater decrease in water intake. Rarely, it may be due to renal disease with impaired ability to excrete sodium
- Hyponatraemia may be due to fluid retention or insufficient sodium, possibly resulting from a poor diet or excess excretion
- Hyperkalaemia can follow from renal failure, acidosis or damaged cells, and can be life-threatening.
- Hypokalaemia may also follow renal disease, but also from gastrointestinal losses, alkalosis and misuse of drugs such as thiazides
- Fluids can be rapidly replaced by IV infusion, but must be adequately monitored and attention paid to renal functioning.

Because the physiology of much of this opening section relies on good kidney function, then this is often presumed, if not demanded. However, this is clearly not always the case and problems with U&Es are often the result of renal disturbances. Therefore we now move on to look at this organ in more detail.

Chapter 7

Investigation of renal function

Key words:

	Normal range
Urea	3.0–8.3 mmol/L
Creatinine	44–133 µol/L
Glomerular filtration rate (GFR)	> 100 ml/min
Uric acid/urate	M < 420, F < 340 µmol/L

Key pathological expressions:

Acute renal failure
Chronic renal failure

An explanation of terms:

Whilst the heart, brain and lungs are the primary concern in emergency care, the kidney is certainly the next organ in importance. This organ consists of millions of single functional units, nephrons (hence nephrology and nephropathy).

Kidney functions

Functions of the kidney

These can be summarised as follows:

- homeostasis: regulating the volume of blood by making urine (diuresis), in maintaining the acid/base balance (i.e., the pH, as may be assessed with hydrogen ions and bicarbonate ions), and in correcting the levels of various electrolytes.
- endocrine activity: regulating blood pressure via local hormones, influencing the bone marrow in the production of red blood cells, and contributing to the level of serum calcium.
- excreting our metabolic waste products, principally the nitrogen-rich molecules urea, uric acid and creatinine.

The top part of the mini-organ of the nephron is the glomerulus – the part that interfaces directly with the blood. It is an important filter: most of the good things in blood pass directly through it, and these are then later re-absorbed so that the leftovers make up the urine. Hence we are interested in the quality of the function of this small area of the nephron.

Glomerular function

Tests of glomerular function

As mentioned, kidney disease is frequently accompanied by changes in U&Es, but especially in serum creatinine and urea. If the former slowly rises up to 150 and beyond to, shall we say, 180, then renal function is deteriorating and the patient is probably in need of a referral to a renal physician. Creatinine itself has few physiological effects – it is most useful as a marker of renal function. However, rising urea is dangerous as it can adversely influence the function of red blood cells and other cells. Levels may also rise because of a decrease in effective circulating blood.

An alternative test of the integrity of this organ is protein in the urine (proteinuria). We all lose a small amount of protein in this way (generally <30 mg in a 24 hour period), and this is physiologically acceptable. Nonetheless, if this loss becomes considerable then renal function must be deteriorating.

However, the ultimate test of kidney function is the rate at which blood is filtered by passing over the glomerulus to produce an early form of urine, i.e. the glomerular filtration rate (GFR). Ideally, this would be about 120 mls/minute, but is accepted to fall slowly with age. In practice, the minimum level for concern is often about 100 mls/minute.

The GFR is calculated by dividing the product of the urine creatinine concentration and 24-hour urine, by the concentration of creatinine in the serum, and so is also known as the creatinine clearance test. The key aspect of this test is the very accurate collection of the 24-hour urine, which must then be sent to the laboratory, along with a sample of serum taken any time within that 24 hours. The laboratory will then do the tests and apply them into the following equation to obtain the GFR:

$$\text{GFR} = \frac{\text{urine concentration of creatinine} \times \text{rate of urine production}}{\text{serum creatinine concentration}}$$

It is hard to over-emphasise that the crucial aspect of this equation is the 24-hour urine. For example, with a urine creatinine concentration of 7.5, a 24-hour urine of 2.16 litres and a serum creatinine of 150, then the GFR should be about 75 mls/minute, which is low.

However, if the 2.16 litres of urine was incorrectly taken over only an 18-hour period, then a true GFR would be about 100, clearly much better and closer to the normal range. Conversely, if only 1.8 litres was collected, instead of the true 2.16 litres, then the GFR would be only 62.5 mls/minute, clearly worse and closer to renal failure. Both these errors could have resulted in starting or withholding crucial therapy.

Overall, therefore, this short example suggests some degree of renal impairment. However, as the serum creatinine was already raised at 150, then this is hardly surprising. Generally, as the creatinine rises, then the GFR falls. At the clinical level, the GFR can fall considerably (such as to 15–20% of normal), and the serum creatinine rises appreciably, before the patient becomes symptomatic.

However, 24-hour urines are being phased out and are not necessarily required for determining the GFR. It can also be calculated from serum creatinine, age, sex and ethnicity.

Renal disease

The aetiology of renal disease

The most common causes of kidney problems can be grouped into three areas (see Figure 7):

- Pre-renal disease is characterised by factors such as insufficient blood entering the kidney, which may be due to occlusive renal artery stenosis, abdominal aortic aneurysm, or poor cardiac output as may be present in heart failure.
- True renal disease is often seen in septic shock, glomerulonephritis (i.e. inflammation of the kidney), in the presence of toxins or amyloid, renal carcinoma (or secondary metastases), and in physical damage with blood loss. This state of the disease may be called acute tubular necrosis.
- Post-renal disease is present if there are problems downstream of the kidney, such as with the ureter, the bladder, or the urethra. Most common causes of this are kidney stones, carcinoma of the bladder or prostate, benign prostatic hyperplasia, or infections. All these limit or prevent urine from flowing out, so that it will eventually back up to the kidneys themselves.

Figure 7 **Aetiology of renal disease**

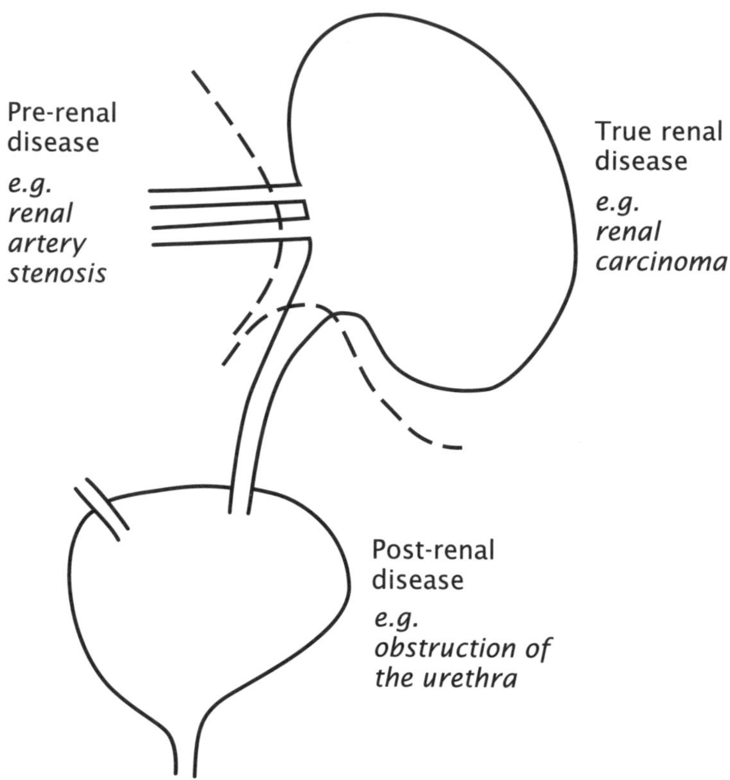

Kidney conditions may be classified as being pre-, true- or post-renal disease. See text for details.

Thus in both pre- and post-renal disease, there is nothing intrinsically wrong with the tissues of the kidney itself, or its functioning: the problem is with the tubes at either end. However, failure to correct pre- or post-renal disease will inevitably lead to acute tubular necrosis. Management of renal disease depends on the particular aetiology and thus the correction of pre/post-renal factors, if appropriate. This may be, for example, antibiotics and immunosuppression for glomerulonephritis, angioplasty for renal artery stenosis, or surgery for bladder carcinoma.

Biochemical monitoring will be by U&Es, and clinically by urine production. If the potassium rises dangerously, then dialysis may well be called for. Recovery from ARF may well be accompanied by a marked diuresis, with a massive increase in urine production (maybe as much as 7 litres a day!), so that fluid balance may need to be checked. Soon after, a return to normal diuresis can be expected.

Acute renal failure

Acute renal failure (ARF)

This may be defined by the ratio of the relative rise in urea being greater than the relative rise in creatinine, not simply the levels themselves. Other biochemical abnormalities include acidosis (because the kidney can no longer excrete hydrogen ions) and hyperkalaemia. Of course, the patient is likely to be able to help in describing any changes in making urine. A likely story is of a sudden fall off, or even cessation, in diuresis.

However, if the damage to the kidney in ARF is excessive, and leads to acute tubular necrosis, it may well become permanently and irreversibly dysfunctional, in which case there will be deterioration to chronic renal failure.

Chronic renal failure

Chronic renal failure (CRF)

CRF is the progressive and (invariably) irreversible destruction of kidney tissues, and is typically noted when the GFR falls below <60 mls/minute. Using U&Es, CRF can be plotted by the relative rise in urea compared to the rise in creatinine. However, unlike ARF, in CRF there is a greater increase in creatinine and a more modest rise in urea.

The consequences of CRF are not unlike those of ARF, principally with disturbances in sodium, hydrogen, and water metabolism – there may be fluid overload or fluid depletion. If present, a metabolic acidosis will be evident with a low level of bicarbonate, and this may also contribute to hyperkalaemia. However, this may independently arise from the increasingly impaired ability to excrete potassium, and may be life-threatening. Low levels of calcium, and hence raised parathyroid hormone (PTH), may be present as the kidney loses its ability to promote calcium absorption in the intestines. Similarly, anaemia is likely to result as the impaired kidney will no longer be making erythropoietin, a growth factor required by those stem cells responsible for red blood cell production.

Clinical features of CRF also include nocturia (resulting from uneven diuresis) and hypertension. Good management will address sodium and water intake, and diuretics may be necessary (depending on the degree of renal (dys)function). Hyperkalaemia may be managed with Resonium A and a low protein diet may help in minimising nitrogen, and thus the need to excrete it as urea and creatinine.

Treatment and care is therefore conservative, and as renal function slowly deteriorates the patient should be prepared physically and psychologically for dialysis, which is generally needed when the GFR falls to about <25 mls/min. The remaining treatment is transplantation.

Urate/ uric acid

Urate/Uric acid: Normal range M <420, F <340 umol/L

Not strictly a marker of renal function, but certainly to do with renal physiology.

Uric acid and its ionised form, urate (dependent on pH), are mostly breakdown products of the synthesis of DNA, and are excreted by the kidney and in the gut. High levels can arise from increased production (maybe 10% of cases) or decreased excretion (perhaps present in 90%). Thus with poor excretion, levels in the blood will rise. Various drugs can also cause an increase in levels of this metabolite.

Urate is particularly insoluble, so that when levels rise they will form crystals (e.g. in the synovial joint) and stones (e.g. in the kidney), leading to further problems such as swelling, pain and inflammation, and ultimately to an arthritis (often gout, where there can also be deposits in the skin). Risk factors for hyper-uricaemia are renal disease, obesity and alcoholism.

Summary of renal function

Summary

- Although urea and creatinine are the cornerstones of the assessment of renal function, we also consider sodium and potassium.
- Increasing levels of potassium can be life-threatening.
- The gold standard test of renal function is the glomerular filtration rate, a test that requires an accurate 24-hour urine collection.
- Acute renal failure (ARF) is often associated with a greater rise in urea than the rise in creatinine.
- Chronic renal failure (CRF) is frequently characterised by a greater rise in creatinine than the rise in urea. There may also be anaemia and hypocalcaemia.
- Renal disease is frequently associated with raised uric acid, and so a gouty arthritis may develop.

Case study 5

A man, aged 75, describes making less and less urine over a period of a few days, and complains to his General Practitioner of something not right 'down there', with occasional pain. The doctor, feeling a hard mass in the lower abdomen, sends a venous sample of blood to the local District General Hospital, with the following results.

	Normal range	**Result**
Na	(133–148)	140
K	(3.3–5.6)	5.4
Urea	(3.0–8.3)	56.5
Creatinine	(44–133)	354

Clue: Compare the rise in urea to the rise in creatinine.

Normal values are also present on page 126.

Interpretation

Abnormal results are raised urea and creatinine, pointing to a problem with the kidney. The increase in urea is about 10 fold over the middle of the normal range, whilst the increase in creatinine is only about 4 times. Thus the relative rise in urea is over twice the relative rise in creatinine, pointing to an initial diagnosis of an acute renal problem. This is supported by the clinical history and anuria.

Diagnosis may be confirmed with imaging (ultrasound) and we can expect a full bladder. A most likely cause of this is blockage of the urethra, maybe by a kidney stone or stones. There seems to be no infection, and a tumour alone would be unlikely to produce such an acute picture.

Chapter 8

Investigation of liver function and plasma proteins

Key words:

	Normal range
Bilirubin	<21 μmol/L
Alkaline phosphatase (Alk Phosp, or ALP)	20–130 IU/L
Gamma glutamyl transpeptidase (Gamma GT)	M<64, F<45 IU/L
Alanine aminotransferase (ALT)	<41 IU/L
Aspartate aminotransferase (AST)	<37 IU/L

Key pathological expressions:

Acute hepatic failure
Cholestasis
Chronic hepatic failure
Hepatitis
Jaundice

An explanation of terms:

Just as a single unit of the kidney is the nephron, a single unit of the liver is a hepatocyte (hence hepatitis [inflammation of the liver] and hepatoma [cancer of the liver], and you can guess from which organ heparin was first purified!). Like the kidney, the liver has a number of functions, but hepatic function is more diverse:

- Metabolic activity of the liver includes synthesis of a large number of different proteins, many destined for 'export' to the blood. Good examples of these are fibrinogen, C-reactive protein (CRP) and the iron transporter transferrin. It is also involved in carbohydrate and lipid metabolism.
- The liver converts glucose and other carbohydrates into the storage compound glycogen, and it also stores iron.

- Detoxification is another important metabolic function, ridding the body of dangerous substances such as plant and animal fungal toxins, paracetamol and alcohol. It is also where pharmaceutical drugs and anaesthetics are broken up and rendered ineffective.

Liver function tests

Liver function tests

When red blood cells come to the end of their life, the proteins and iron in haemoglobin are recycled, but certain complex molecules (for example, bilirubin) are not. The precise biochemistry of the family of molecules is complex and beyond the scope of this text. Bilirubin, often carried by albumin, finds its way to the liver where it is excreted via the gall bladder, bile duct and so into the intestines. Thus if the liver is unable to perform this function, the level of bilirubin in the blood rises.

The liver synthesises and then exports a large number of proteins into the blood. So if the levels of these proteins, such as albumin, fibrinogen and prothrombin, fall, we consider failure of production. Alternatively, low levels may arise from excess consumption. However, another explanation for low levels is malnutrition, so jumping to conclusions can be dangerous!

Enzymes involved in biosynthesis and metabolism include the aminotransferases alanine aminotransferase (ALT) and aspartate aminotransferase (AST), alkaline phosphatase (Alk Phos, or ALP) and gamma glutamyl transferase (Gamma GT, or GGT). Between them, these enzymes are the tools the liver cells use to break up large molecules into their component parts, and then use some of these parts to synthesise new molecules. Un-used parts are excreted (for example, as urea and creatinine).

However, a big problem with these enzymes is that they are not specific for the liver. Substantial amounts of alkaline phosphatase are present in the bone, small intestine, placenta and kidney. Gamma GT is also widely distributed, being present in the kidney and pancreas. This enzyme is also sensitive to alcohol and certain drugs, such as phenytoin. AST and ALT are also widely distributed, being present in skeletal and cardiac muscle and in the kidney, although ALT is more liver-specific. Hence AST may be raised following myocardial infarction.

Although strictly not a liver function test, now is a good time to mention alpha-feto protein (AFP) as it is raised in 80–90% of primary liver cancers (hepatoma). Levels are generally not raised when the liver carries metastatic cells from a distant primary tumour. Liver cancers, of whatever aetiology, generally display raised gamma GT, alkaline phosphatase and bilirubin.

Jaundice

Jaundice

This clinical sign is characterised by a yellow colouring, most evident in the sclera of the eye, and is caused by high serum bilirubin, generally greater than 40 μmol/L. So there is a large gap between the top end of the normal range (21 μmol/L) and the most common presenting (visual) sign. However, people with a developing jaundice often have abdominal discomfort, lack of appetite, lethargy, tiredness and general non-specific illness for several days before the jaundice becomes evident. The aetiology of jaundice is most variable.

Liver disease

Types of Liver Disease

As with renal disease, we can consider pre-, true, and post-liver disease.

- As mentioned, when red blood cells come to the end of their lifespan they are removed from the circulation and broken up. The un-recycled part, bilirubin, remains in the blood and is eventually cleared, mostly by the liver, and some by the kidney. However, if there is excessive haemolysis, then the liver is unable to keep up purifying the blood of the high levels of bilirubin, then levels rise and can cause jaundice. Thus there is nothing intrinsically wrong with the liver itself, it just can't keep up with the high levels of bilirubin resulting from excessive red cell destruction.
- True damage to the hepatocyte (i.e. hepatocellular damage) is often seen in, for example, cases of poisoning by inhaled solvents in paint spray, or in viral hepatitis. This would initially be characterised biochemically by increases in aminotransferases ALT and AST, and later by rising bilirubin as the excretory function of the liver is influenced.
- A good example of post-hepatic disease is obstruction or stenosis of the bile duct by factors such as gall stones, or inflammation or tumour of the head of the bile duct or pancreatic duct (cholestasis). Thus, again, the initial problem is not the tissue of the liver itself, but with the associated plumbing. However, as with pre- and post-renal disease, failure to act on pre- and post-liver disease will eventually lead to true liver disease.

Figure 8 **Aetiology of liver disease**

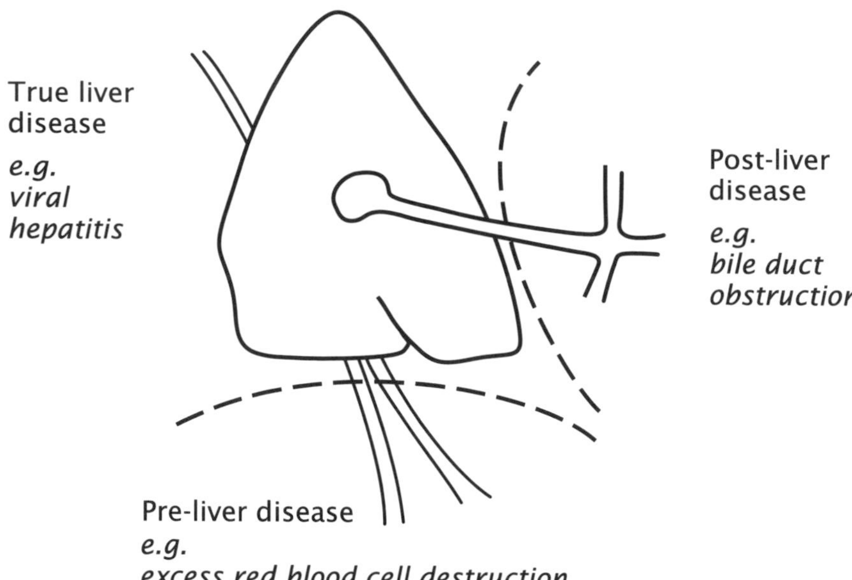

Liver conditions may be classified as being pre-, true- or post-hepatic disease. See the text for details

Acute liver disease

Acute liver disease

Almost by definition, onset is rapid and can generally be ascribed to a single factor or event. Poisoning (e.g. organic solvents, carbon tetrachloride), drug overdose (e.g. barbiturates, herbicides), shock, severe hypoxia and acute cardiac failure are good examples of factors that precipitate acute disease. In such cases, rising levels of AST and ALT are frequently seen, followed maybe days later by bilirubin. An alternative scenario is sudden blockage of the bile duct by a stone (i.e. cholestasis). This would be more likely to be characterised by rising alkaline phosphatase and gamma GT. In some cases, viral hepatitis can be traced to a precise (infective) event.

Chronic liver disease

Chronic liver disease

Again, by definition, we suspect a slow and insidious disease process, although it may also have a precise defining event, and can follow from acute disease. For example, a hepatitis virus infection may be partially treated in the short term, with a modest return of normal liver function, but chronic active hepatitis may result. A further example is cholestasis resulting from a slowly developing blockage, such as a tumour, which the surgeons may be able to treat, although, like chronic renal failure, the chronic liver disease is generally irreversible.

Other common causes of chronic liver disease are alcoholism and the auto-immune disease primary biliary cirrhosis. However, whatever the aetiology, the laboratory notes rising plasma markers of liver function, although in the terminal stages levels of some will fall as the liver is unable to synthesise them: hence a risk of bleeding due to insufficient clotting proteins. Bilirubin will continue to rise and can be treated by dialysis, although this is clearly only palliative. The only effective treatment is transplantation, although this is, of course, by no means 100% successful.

A Cautionary Tale – 2

Several months after marriage, a young woman developed an irreversibly rapid and fulminant jaundice that progressed to liver failure and so death. The husband subsequently remarried, only to find his second wife suffering almost exactly the same fate. The unfortunate widower identified a third possible spouse, but during their courtship she also became jaundiced, although this time the hepatitis was not fatal.

Investigations into the man found him to be an asymptomatic hepatitis B virus carrier with all liver function tests mildly abnormal. Although clearly (with hindsight) inoculating his three sexual partners with semen loaded with hepatitis B virus, the compassionate nature of the case was clear and the authorities decided against charging him with manslaughter.

From a letter to a learned Journal during the 1980s
(with apologies to the author and editor)

Plasma proteins

Key words:

	Normal range
Total protein	63–84 g/L
Albumin	35–50 g/L
Prostate specific antigen (PSA)	< 6.5 μg/L, but age dependent
C-reactive protein (CRP)	< 5 mg/L
Amylase	< 110 IU/L

Key pathological expressions:

Hypoalbuminaemia
Inflammation

An explanation of terms:

The laboratory offers total plasma proteins, and albumin, the latter generally making up about half of all the proteins. The remaining half is made up of dozens of other proteins (such as CRP, immunoglobulins and PSA), all at different individual concentrations. Many tumour markers are proteins.

Total proteins

As mentioned above, this global score assesses all plasma proteins. Raised total proteins can therefore (in theory) be due to any individual protein, although in practice the only protein to do this is increased levels of immunoglobulins as may be present in an infection, or in a myeloma. Decreased total protein is almost always due to hypoalbuminaemia.

Albumin

This molecule is important for a number of reasons, e.g. being a carrier of calcium, bilirubin and various other substances. Low levels of albumin will therefore have other consequences. Another indication of the importance of albumin is in the maintenance of tissue fluid: low albumin will be a contributing factor in oedema. Hypoalbuminaemia may be due to poor liver function, as almost all arises in the liver, or in cases of inadequate nutrition or malabsorption, overhydration, or severe nephrotic syndrome, where kidney damage is so great that albumin is lost in the urine.

C-reactive protein

C-reactive protein (CRP)

This marker of inflammation, like ESR, is typically raised in autoimmune diseases, and in bacterial infections. It will therefore often go together with a raised WBCC. Produced by the liver by the same process as causes pyrexia, it is frequently described as an acute phase protein.

The remaining 50% or so of the total plasma protein pool is made up of numerous proteins, many of which we have already come across. These are listed in Table 5. Amylase is likely to be raised in pancreatitis and pancreatic cancer.

Functions of plasma protein

Table 5

Functions of plasma proteins

Protein	function
Transferrin	iron transport
Fibrinogen	coagulation
Amylase	pancreatic digestive enzyme
Insulin	glucoregulatory hormone
Cancer markers	**cancer marked:**
Prostate specific antigen (PSA)	prostate
Alpha-feto protein (AFP)	liver
CA-125	ovary
Immunoglobulins	myeloma

Summary

Summary of liver function tests and plasma proteins

- The aetiology of liver disease, like that of the kidney, considers pre-, true- and post-hepatic causes.
- LFTs include alkaline phosphate, bilirubin, gamma GT, ALT and AST. They are used to diagnose and investigate conditions such as jaundice.
- Common causes of acute liver disease include cholestasis and viral hepatitis. Chronic liver disease often arises from alcoholism, primary biliary cirrhosis, or from acute (long-standing) hepatic damage.
- Total proteins and albumin are also important in assessing liver function. Low levels may be due to impaired synthesis and/or malnutrition.
- Many plasma proteins have identifiable functions as hormones, enzymes, or as cancer markers.

Case study 6

A male, aged 68, reports being increasingly tired and lethargic over a six months period, with weight loss, despite his wife's attempts to 'feed him up'. More recently, he complains of abdominal discomfort. Blood results are as follows (normal values in brackets):

Na	(133–148)	138	**K**	(3.3–5.6)	4.0
Urea	(3.0–8.3)	6.1	**Creatinine**	(44–133)	89
Total Protein	(63–84)	60	**Albumin**	(35–50)	28
Alk phosphatase	(20–130)	190	**AST**	(<37)	89
Bilirubin	(<21)	22	**ALT**	(<41)	72
Gamma GT	(<64)	215			
Fibrinogen	(1.5–4.0)	1.3	**Amylase**	(<110)	25
CRP	(<5)	2.0	**ESR**	(<10)	15

Interpretation

There are no abnormalities in the tests of renal function, so we can discount problems in this organ. However, all five liver function tests are abnormal, so this organ is clearly under suspicion. We also have a low fibrinogen and abnormal ESR but normal amylase and CRP. The abnormalities in fibrinogen, with low total protein and albumin also indicate liver dysfunction, but the raised ESR provides little extra help. No increase in CRP points to a lack of an on-going inflammatory response.

Additional tests would include hepatitis virus screening (A, B and C), with ultrasound imaging to check the integrity of the gall bladder. Since there is an ESR result then we presume there must be a full blood count somewhere. If not, it should certainly be ordered. The immunology laboratory will help with considering primary biliary cirrhosis. Additional questions to the patient may reveal use of alcohol (although, of course, this may not always be reliable). A liver biopsy may help, although this may be dangerous in view of low coagulation proteins.

Chapter 9

Atherosclerosis and its risk factors

This chronic condition, characterised by damage to the blood vessel wall followed by thrombosis and hypertension, is likely to strike the majority of the Western World. The late stages, stroke, myocardial infarction and critical limb ischaemia (of the leg) are almost always preceded by warning signs of transient ischaemic attack, angina, and intermittent claudication. However, more pertinently, clinical disease is generally preceded by well-known risk factors: diabetes, smoking, hypertension and hypercholesterolaemia. There are no direct routine laboratory tests in hypertension, but some tests can assess smoking status, although the laboratory is likely to resist such a request. The laboratory is helpful in the diagnosis of diabetes and hyperlipidaemia, and in the monitoring of treatment.

Diabetes mellitus

Diabetes mellitus

Key words:

	Normal range
Fasting plasma glucose	< 6.1 mmol/L
Oral glucose tolerance test (OGTT)	Two hour peak glucose < 7.8 mmol/L
Glycosylated haemoglobin (HbA1c)	3.3–5.5 %

Key pathological expressions:

Diabetes mellitus
Diabetic ketoacidosis
Hyperglycaemia
Impaired fasting glycaemia
Impaired glucose tolerance

An explanation of terms:

This condition can arise without an obvious cause (i.e. primary) or may be secondary to factors such as obesity, drugs, pancreatic disease or Cushing's syndrome. It is the most common endocrine disorder, characterised by hyperglycaemia due to lack or dysfunction of insulin. Indeed, as of 2000, there were 1,466,800 people in the UK known to have diabetes. Complete lack of insulin leads to insulin dependent diabetes mellitus (IDDM, about 15% of diabetics, often occurring in the young), whilst insulin resistance is the basis of non-insulin dependent diabetes mellitus (NIDDM, making up 85%, generally arising in later life and associating with obesity). As more than 50% of adults are overweight (e.g. body mass index greater than 25) then there is a considerable amount of occult or pre-diabetes.

The pathology of diabetes is established: in the early stages there is hyperglycaemia with symptoms such as polyuria, polydipsia and weight loss. This leads to microvascular disease (retinopathy, neuropathy and nephropathy) and then to atherosclerosis, characterised symptomatically by coronary artery disease. Naturally, there is great variety in presenting symptoms and rate of progression from person to person.

Blood glucose

Blood glucose

N.b. blood glucose is perhaps the only routine biochemistry blood test that is not performed on clotted blood and needs to be taken into the anti-coagulant FLOX (check with your laboratory).

Because glucose levels in the blood vary considerably during the day, the timing of the blood test is crucial, with lowest levels in the morning before eating breakfast. Hence the importance of a FASTING sample. The alternative is a random sample. Therefore random and fasting samples are very different and so have different normal (target) ranges. Plasma levels also give different results from whole blood levels, so that blood from the vein is different from capillary blood from a fingerprick. A fasting glucose of less than 6.1 mmol/L is to be expected from non-diabetics. However, for a complete diagnosis, an oral glucose tolerance test is also performed.

OGTT

The oral glucose tolerance test (OGTT)

A better method of checking a preliminary diagnosis of diabetes is with the OGTT. Here, the fasted subject arrives at the laboratory at perhaps 9.00 a.m., gives a blood sample, and then drinks 75g of glucose. Additional blood samples can be obtained every hour up to 3 hours, and levels of glucose in the blood are plotted. However, many laboratories dispense with repeated samples, and often simply take a baseline and 2-hour sample. A healthy response sees levels rise to a peak of less than 7.8 mmol/L at 2 hours, after which time levels fall. The response of a diabetic will be increasing glucose from a high fasting level (i.e. greater than 6.1) that rises to peak at over 11 mmol/L and then a fall, although levels may not even peak after two hours in the most unregulated cases. Such a response is required on two separate occasions for a firm diagnosis of diabetes.

Figure 9

The oral glucose tolerance test: typical profiles

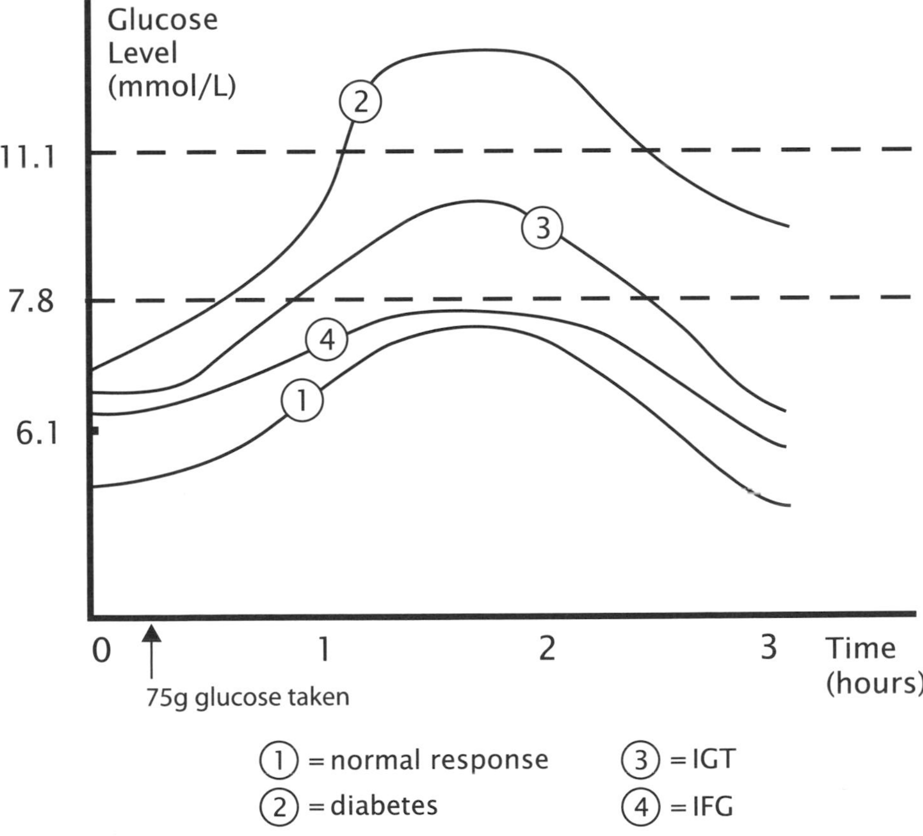

However, some results do not fall into either of these scenarios. One patient's samples may rise rapidly, and exceed the magic 11 mmol/L, but then fall rapidly back into the normal range. Alternatively, another's may rise slowly, never exceed 11 mmol/L, but scarcely fall at all (figure 9). These and other data demand expert interpretation, and tentative diagnoses of impaired glucose tolerance (IGT) and impaired fasting glycaemia (IFG) may be offered. These are certainly not diabetes, but could be a risk factor for classical diabetes at some time in the future. Therefore regular monitoring is required.

- IGT may be defined as a fasting glucose less than 7.0 mmol/L *and* a 2 hours glucose between 7.7 and 11.1 mmol/L.
- IFG may be defined by a fasting glucose between 6.0 and 7.0 mmol/L *and* a 2 hour result less than 7.8 mmol/L.

Glycosylated haemoglobin

Glycosylated haemoglobin (HbA1c)

Hyperglycaemia is not benign: it is not simply a situation of too much sugar in the blood. High sugar sticks to other proteins and cells and influences their function. One such interaction is with the haemoglobin within red blood cells, some proportion of which binds the glucose, hence is described as glycosylated haemoglobin, called in the laboratory HbA1c. As the glucose stays on the haemoglobin, then it remains there for the entire life of that red cell. Consequently, increased HbA1c indicates poor long-term control of the hyperglycaemia, and as such is useful in checking the effect of treatment over a 3 month period.

Diabetic ketoacidosis

Diabetic ketoacidosis (DKA)

This clinical situation is found in cases of severe hyperglycaemia, and represents probably the most important crisis a diabetic can face. It is characterised by a cycle of insulin resistance and/or deficiency, with hyperglycaemia, acidosis and dehydration. Pathophysiologically, two overlapping cycles exist.

The first centres on hyperglycaemia, which invariably leads to glycosuria. It is not enough simply to excrete glucose in urine – it must be excreted with a great deal of water (thus the symptoms of polyuria) leading eventually to dehydration. The consequences of loss of blood volume include hypotension, shock and pre-renal uraemia resulting from a fall in the glomerular filtration rate. This, in turn, leads, via several complex hormones and factors, to insulin deficiency and/or resistance, thus back to hyperglycaemia.

Changes in the 'several complex hormones and factors' also lead to the second part of the cycle. These, alongside insulin problems, can lead to changes in lipid metabolism and the mobilisation of fatty acids from adipose tissues into the blood. Ketone bodies rise, and these can lead to acidosis with an associated hyperkalaemia. This promotes nausea and then vomiting, and so loss of fluids and eventual dehydration.

The laboratory can help in diagnosis, investigation and treatment of DKA. There are various opportunities to intervene in this cycle, with intravenous fluids to treat dehydration, and insulin to get glucose out of the blood and into cells. This hormone will also help the hyperkalaemia. If the acidosis is severe, then a bicarbonate drip can be used, which may also help address the high potassium.

Hypo-glycaemia

Hypoglycaemia

Defined by a glucose level less than 2.8 mmol/L, 99% of hypoglycaemic attacks are in patients with IDDM. Cognitive disturbances are common when levels fall below 2.0 mmol/L, followed by ECG changes, coma and death. Causes include reduced intake of carbohydrates, over-use of insulin, excess exercise or excess consumption of alcohol. Treatments include oral glucose, chocolate-rich confectionary or jam, or intra-muscular injections of the hormone glucagon. However, if the patient is unconscious intravenous glucose or dextrose will be required.

Hyperlipidaemia

Hyper-lipidaemia

Key words:

	Normal (target) range
Total cholesterol	2.5–5.0 mmol/L
HDL-cholesterol	> 1.0 mmol/L
Triglycerides	< 2.3 mmol/L

Key pathological expressions:

Hypercholesterolaemia
Hypertriglyceridaemia

An explanation of terms:

The two major classes of lipids are cholesterol and triglycerides. As with diabetes, hypercholesterolaemia can be primary and secondary: the latter may be due to a poor (fat-rich) diet (with or without obesity), hypothyroidism, alcoholism, chronic renal failure or, indeed, to diabetes itself. The most common primary cause of raised lipids is genetic. Familial hypercholesterolaemia is the most common, but there are others, including familial hypertriglycerid-aemia (raised triglycerides) and familial combined hyperlipidaemia (raised cholesterol and triglycerides).

Knowledge of serum cholesterol is necessary to be able to assess the risk of developing symptomatic atherosclerosis. Although total cholesterol is a good guide to risk, a sub-fraction, LDL-cholesterol, is more accurate. Unfortunately, LDL-cholesterol is very difficult to measure directly, but can be worked out according to a formula that consists of total cholesterol, HDL-cholesterol and triglycerides. Like glucose, levels of triglycerides can vary throughout the day so that fasting levels are necessary for the most precise assessment. Should it be needed, the relevant equation for LDL is:

$$\text{LDL-cholesterol} = \text{total cholesterol} - \text{HDL-cholesterol} - \frac{(\text{triglycerides})}{2.19}$$

However, this equation is only applicable to triglyceride levels less than 3.0 mmol/L. Of course, someone at risk of hypercholestero-laemia may well also be at risk of diabetes – so that at the same time a fasting glucose sample may as well also be taken.

High levels of total and LDL-cholesterol, and low HDL-cholesterol, are important as predictors of cardiovascular disease, but they are not, of course, the only such predictors – others include increasing age, male sex, smoking, diabetes, and left ventricular hypertrophy. These factors can be entered into a complex formula that hopes to predict and thus identify those at high risk of an adverse event (heart attack or stroke) in, shall we say, the next ten years. Lipid-lowering therapy, such as a statin, can then be more accurately targeted.

Coronary Atherosclerosis

Coronary athero-sclerosis

Key words:

	Normal range
Creatine kinase (CK)	< 150 IU/L (higher in Afro-Caribbeans)
CK-MB	< 25 IU/L
Troponin T	Low risk < 0.1 ng/mL, high risk > 0.6 ng/mL

Key pathological expressions:

Angina
Myocardial infarction

An explanation of terms:

There are no specific laboratory tests for the presence of cerebrovascular disease (stroke), or atherosclerotic disease of the legs (as may be suggested by intermittent claudication and critical limb ischaemia). However, there are tests for the consequences of atherosclerosis of the coronary arteries as is very likely to be present following a myocardial infarction. These are as follows:

- The heart is simply a modified muscle, so that enzymes present in damaged muscle can be expected to be raised after a heart attack. Such an enzyme is creatine kinase (CK). However, CK is also present in skeletal muscle, so that raised levels may also arise from damage to these tissues, such as may be present following heavy exercise (like running a marathon!) or in the muscle disease polymyositis. Therefore raised levels can only strictly be used with an appropriate history (chest pain etc.) and ECG changes.
- CK-MB is a variant of total CK that is more specific for heart muscle, so therefore may be more useful.
- An even more specific marker is troponin T, another is troponin I. These are not enzymes but actual heart muscle protein, and so are of even more precise specificity. However, Table 6 provides examples of conditions where there are raised levels in the absence of a heart attack.

The value of these markers has to be weighed against the time course of the reaction to the myocardial infarction: the markers' response at different times, troponins being the slowest (6–12hr) to peak. Marker use is compounded by the differences in the time that the patients present to hospital after their infarction: some will present immediately, others hours later.

Other serum markers include myoglobin and lactate dehydrogenase although, like hydroxyl-butyrate dehydrogenase, these may or may not pass the test of time. 'Liver' enzymes such as alanine and aspartate aminotransferases may also rise after an acute myocardial infarction.

Raised troponins

Table 6
Indications of raised troponins

Cardiac disease and interventions
Cardiac amyloidosis, cardiac contusion, cardiac surgery, cardioversion and implantable cardioverter defibrillator shocks, closure of atrial septal defects, coronary vasospasm, dilated cardiomyopathy, heart failure, hypertrophic cardiomyopathy, myocarditis, percutaneous coronary intervention, post-cardiac transplantation, radiofrequency ablatation, supraventricular tachycardia,

Non-cardiac diseases
Critically ill patients, high dose chemotherapy, primary pulmonary hypertension, pulmonary embolism, renal failure, subarachnoid haemorrhage, scorpion envenoming, sepsis and septic shock, stroke, ultra-endurance exercise (marathon).

Source: *British Medical Journal* 2004, 328: 1028–9.
Issue of 1st May 2004.

Summary

Summary of atherosclerosis and its risk factors

- There are no laboratory tests specific for hypertension: the laboratory is most unlikely to agree to test for smoking.
- Diabetes can be diagnosed and monitored with fasting glucose and HbA1c; the oral glucose tolerance test is also useful, especially in clarifying the diagnosis and considering impaired glucose tolerance and impaired fasting glycaemia.
- Total cholesterol and HDL-cholesterol can be measured on a random sample; LDL-cholesterol is calculated from a formula that demands a fasting triglyceride.
- Creatine kinase (CK), CK-MB and troponins are used to help diagnose myocardial infarction

Chapter 10

Calcium, bone and musculo-skeletal disease

Key words:

	Normal range
Calcium	2.2–2.6 mmol/L
Parathyroid hormone (PTH)	10–65 pg/mL
Albumin	35–50 g/L
Alkaline phosphatase	20–130 IU/L
Phosphate	0.81–1.45 mmol/L
Creatine kinase	< 150 IU/mL

Key pathological expressions:

Hypercalcaemia
Hypocalcaemia

An explanation of terms:

Calcium

Calcium

This is the most abundant mineral in the body, and 99% of it is in bone. In the blood it is regulated by parathyroid hormone (PTH) acting on different tissues to raise circulating levels by increasing absorption across the gut wall, by minimising excretion, and by mobilising bone stores. PTH arises from the parathyroid glands that are stimulated to produce and release PTH by a releasing factor. Low levels of blood calcium are detected and the releasing factor secreted by the combined action of the pituitary and hypothalamus. As plasma calcium levels rise this secretion is switched off – a classic example of feedback regulation.

About half of our plasma calcium circulates bound to albumin, and it is the unbound balance, known as 'free' or ionised calcium, which the pituitary and hypothalamus respond to. This process is pH dependent, so that in acidosis the ionised calcium increases and conversely at an alkalotic pH, it falls. Consequently, in acute respiratory alkalosis, tetany may occur due to the sudden decrease in ionised calcium. The laboratory measures total calcium, i.e. free and bound, so that interpretation is required. If albumin is low, total calcium may be low as a result, but the free calcium will frequently be satisfactory. Thus such a situation is not true hypocalcaemia. If there is indeed low (total) calcium and low albumin, then a calculation is required. This is:

Adjusted calcium = Total calcium + [0.02 (40 - albumin concentration)]

The Path Lab will do this calculation, so there is no need to memorise it! Thus adjusted calcium may well move into the normal range, so reducing concern.

Like almost all analytes, we consider the implications of levels above and below the normal range.

Hyper-calcaemia

Hypercalcaemia

Present in perhaps 5% of in-patients, most cases of high plasma calcium (i.e. >2.6 mmol/L) can be explained by a small number of causes:

- Primary hyperparathyroidism results in high levels of PTH (>53pg/mL) that in turn cause the high blood calcium levels. This, in turn, may result from a tumour of the parathyroid gland that secretes PTH regardless of instruction from the pituitary and hypothalamus.
- Malignancy: most often a tumour secreting a PTH-like protein, or else a tumour (such as a myeloma or secondaries from a breast carcinoma) that has invaded and mobilises bone to make more space for itself, resulting in calcium release from bone and its movement into the blood. In such a case there may well be low or normal PTH levels.
- Rare reasons for high calcium include excess calcium intake, immobilisation, thyroid disease, renal disease, and inappropriate use of vitamin D, diuretics and lithium.

Since calcium is important in nerve conduction, treatment is urgent if levels exceed 3.5 mmol/L, as cardiac arrhythmias, and then arrest may follow. Treatments include vigorous rehydration, a drug from the bis-phosphonate family (especially in myeloma), calcitonin and prednisolone. However, the original cause of the problem must eventually be addressed (e.g. surgical excision of a PTH-secreting adenoma).

Hypo-calcaemia

Hypocalcaemia

Recall that low calcium (< 2.2 mmol/L) by itself is not necessarily true hypocalcaemia: it may be related to a low albumin and adjusted calcium may rise to be within the normal range. Investigation centres on abnormal intake and regulation:

- Hypoparathyroidism resulting from failure of the parathyroid gland, possibly due to autoimmune disease or the excesses of treatments for hyperthyroidism, such as over-use of radio-active iodine or poor surgical technique.
- Renal disease: (a) this organ secretes a molecule essential for absorption of calcium from the intestines (i.e. secondary malabsorption), (b) damage to the nephron so that calcium is not re-absorbed from the developing urine and is thus excreted.
- Inadequate intake of calcium and/or vitamin D in the diet.

Like hypercalcaemia, clinical features include an abnormal ECG, and treatment must address the cause(s). Oral supplements are one avenue, synthetic vitamin D analogues another. If urgent, a calcium supplement may be added to an intravenous drip

Phosphate

Phosphate

About 85% of body phosphate is in the bone, and there is a marked diurnal effect. Levels are often reciprocal with calcium. The commonest form of hyperphosphataemia is renal failure (reduced excretion), others are hypoparathyroidism and cell lysis. Severe hypophosphataemia (< 0.3, possibly due to raised PTH) is rare, causes muscle weakness, may lead to respiratory failure, and demands urgent treatment with intravenous supplements. Other causes include treatment of diabetic ketoacidosis with insulin (as the shift of glucose into the cell may cause a similar movement of phosphates) and alkalosis.

Bone disease

Bone disease

Contrary to popular belief, measurement of calcium usually has little to offer the bone disease that has the highest profile – osteoporosis – although oral calcium supplements as a treatment have been advocated. Similarly, Paget's disease is rarely characterised by abnormal calcium or phosphates but a raised alkaline phosphatase is a frequent finding, indicating increased bone turnover, and may also be raised in hyperparathyroidism and metastatic cancer.

Musculo-skeletal disease

Musculo-skeletal disease

This group includes auto-immune conditions such as rheumatoid arthritis, systemic lupus erythematosus, systemic sclerosis/ scleroderma and ankylosing spondylitis. There are no routine blood tests for these conditions, but the laboratory can pass blood on to a specialist laboratory (often an Immunology Lab.) for rheumatoid factor, anti-nuclear antibodies, complement and for HLA-B27 testing. However, as these diseases often have an inflammatory component, white blood cell count and CRP may be ordered.

As elsewhere, the laboratory provides guidance on diagnosis and the effects of treatment. This is particularly pertinent as many of these diseases are inflammatory, and so we hope particular immunosuppressive treatments will improve laboratory markers of inflammation such as ESR. The effects of steroids on giant cell arteritis are an example of the use of this marker.

Recall that creatine kinase may also be produced by non-cardiac muscle, so may be increased in conditions such as polymyositis, and can also be increased by the use of certain drugs (statins) designed to lower cholesterol.

Summary of calcium, bone and musculo-skeletal disease

Summary

- Almost all body calcium and phosphate is in bone: in the plasma they have a reciprocal relationship.
- Plasma calcium levels are regulated by feedback inhibition by PTH.
- Hypercalcaemia may be driven by inappropriately high levels of PTH or mobilisation of bone stores by a malignancy.
- Hypocalcaemia must first be checked for a low albumin, and then, if necessary, adjusted. Otherwise, it may be due to failure of PTH, poor diet, or renal disease.
- Marked hypercalcaemia demands urgent action.
- The laboratory is unable to help in most bone conditions, except Paget's disease, where raised alkaline phosphatase alone is a frequent finding.
- There are no specific or routine tests for musculo-skeletal disorders, but several tests can help provide a direction.

Case study 7

A 65-year-old woman complains of being increasingly tired and lethargic over a period of several months. Her family doctor sends a blood sample to the Pathology Laboratory of the local District General Hospital. Results were as follows:

Na	(133–148)	149	**K**	(3.3–5.6)	4.3
Urea	(3.0–8.3)	11.3	**Creatinine**	(44–133)	708
T Protein	(63–84)	65	**Albumin**	(35–50)	33
Calcium	(2.2–2.6)	1.8	**Alk phosphatase**	(20–130)	231
Bilirubin	(<21)	12	**Alanine AT**	(<41)	35
Gamma GT	(<45)	55	**Glucose**	(<6.1)	4.5

Figures in brackets are the normal range.

Interpretation

Sodium is very slightly raised, probably not enough to warrant a great deal of concern. However, there is marginally raised urea (twice the middle of the normal range) with considerably raised creatinine (about 6-fold). The increase in creatinine is much greater than the increase in urea, a result suggesting chronic renal failure. Also present is low albumin, low calcium and raised alkaline phosphatase.

Application of the calcium result into the adjustment equation gives a corrected value of 2.1, so that the hypocalcaemia, although very mild, may be real. If so, it may be due to hypoparathyroidism (demanding measurement of PTH), or to low dietary calcium and vitamin D, or to renal disease, something we already have. Raised alkaline phosphatase but no other abnormalities in LFTs implies an extra-hepatic origin, such as bone, intestine or the kidney. Thus the treatment path first addresses the renal problem, which may in turn result in an improvement in calcium. Whilst ordering additional bloods, a full blood count may be worthwhile to look for a possible anaemia

Chapter 11

Investigation of thyroid function

Key words:

	Normal range
Free thyroxine (T4)	10–24 pmol/L
Thyroid stimulating hormone (TSH)	0.4–5.5 mIU/L

Key pathological expressions:

Thyroiditis
Thyroxotoxicosis

An explanation of terms:

As the thyroid hormones (T3 and T4) are required for the correct regulation of a host of maturational and metabolic pathways (such as of lipids), then very many clinical symptoms and laboratory changes follow from abnormal levels. Almost all (99%) of the body's mass of these hormones are transported by plasma proteins, including albumin, hence measurement of free T4 (i.e. that amount unbound by carrier proteins).

Like calcium, levels of thyroid hormones are regulated by feedback via the pituitary and hypothalamus, that together release TSH to instruct the thyroid to make more T3 and T4. Indeed, maybe 10% of patients also have hypercalcaemia. Thus, in theory, if thyroid hormones are low, then TSH should be high in order to prompt the thyroid to increase synthesis. Conversely, if levels of T3 and T4 are adequate, then TSH should not be needed and so levels will be low. Most laboratories will offer T4 and TSH, arguing that measurement of T3 generally offers little extra, although T3 can be useful in some cases of hyperthyroidism.

Iodine is a major component of T3 and T4, and insufficient dietary iodine can cause the thyroid to swell, resulting in a goitre. However, goitre may also be due to a tumour.

Hyper-thyroidism

Hyperthyroidism

Present in perhaps 1 % of the general population, diagnosis of this condition, also known as thyrotoxicosis, is by high T4 and low TSH. However, there are instances of normal T4 but raised T3 in some cases of hyperthyroidism.

High levels of T4 can arise from autoimmune disease (such as Graves disease, the most common cause), adenoma or generalised inflammation of the thyroid (i.e. thyroiditis). Rarely, a tumour of the pituitary/hypothalamus will over-stimulate the thyroid by producing unregulated excess TSH. Amiodarone, used to treat atrial fibrillation, also causes thyrotoxicosis in 3–5 % of patients.

Treatments include anti-thyroid dugs (e.g. carbimazole, that may also cause neutropenia, thus illustrating the close relationship between biochemistry and haematology), radioactive iodine, and surgery. Thyroid function tests are essential in monitoring these treatments.

Hypo-thyroidism

Hypothyroidism

Diagnosis also relies on T4 and TSH, but in the reverse, i.e. low T4 with high TSH. Most cases of hypothyroidism result from destruction or failure of the thyroid gland by autoimmune mechanisms or over-treatment of hyperthyroidism. A rare cause is failure of the pituitary/hypothalamus to produce TSH.

Whatever the aetiology, treatment is with thyroxine, and its effect (or lack of) on the thyroid is monitored with blood tests.

Summary of thyroid function tests

Summary

- The laboratory generally offers free T4 and TSH
- Hyperthyroidism is most often characterised by high T4 and low TSH
- Hypothyroidism is generally associated with low T4 but high TSH

Chapter 12

Blood Gases and pH

Key words:

	Normal range
Hydrogen ions (H^+)	36–44 nmol/L
pH	7.36–7.44
Bicarbonate (HCO_3^-)	24–32 mmol/L
Blood carbon dioxide (PCO_2)	4.5–6.1 kPa
Blood oxygen (PO_2)	12–15 kPa

Key pathological expressions:

Metabolic acidosis
Metabolic alkalosis
Respiratory acidosis
Respiratory alkalosis

An explanation of terms:

The *P* in PO_2 and PCO_2 indicates partial pressure. Rarely, total CO_2 may be requested, being the sum of dissolved CO_2, carbonic acid and bicarbonate. However, 95% of this total value is contributed by the bicarbonate. PO_2 is often used to monitor the efficiency of oxygen therapy. In blood gas analysis, the bicarbonate is not measured directly but is calculated from the H^+ and the PCO_2 alone, in contrast to 'normal' serum biochemistry, where bicarbonate is measured directly.

As we have discussed, the waste products of our normal metabolism include urea and creatinine, to which we can now add hydrogen ions (H^+) and carbon dioxide (CO_2). The former is excreted in urine, the latter at the lungs in our exhaled breath. It follows that disease in either organ will lead to changes in these blood components. Levels of H^+ being too high, and thus the pH being low (tending to, or lower than, pH 7), is acidosis. Conversely, when the pH is high (tending to, or exceeding pH 7.6), with low levels of H^+, there is likely to be alkalosis. However, the picture is complex and therefore requires some explanation.

Hydrogen ions can exist by themselves or as part of water, and increased H^+ leads to a low pH and acidosis. However, CO_2 is part of the system as it can combine with water to give carbonic acid, in the following equation:

$$H_2O + CO_2 = H_2CO_3$$

This indeed is how a great deal of carbon dioxide is carried from the tissues to the lungs in red blood cells. The carbonic acid, acting as a weak acid, can itself break down to a hydrogen ion and the bicarbonate ion:

$$H_2CO_3 = H^+ + HCO_3^-$$

The regulation (homeostasis) of this system is quite robust and various checks and balances are in place (mostly in the kidney) to ensure the status quo is maintained. For example, there are various buffer systems (such as bicarbonate, phosphate, haemoglobin and proteins) designed to keep the level of H^+ acceptable. So if the level of H^+ falls, more can be generated from carbonic acid. When carbonic acid itself runs low, more can be generated from water and carbon dioxide.

When this system breaks down, the result is acidosis or alkalosis. The primary pathology can depend on respiratory disorders where the primary pulmonary defect in ventilation affects the PCO_2. An alternative is a metabolic disorder, of which there may be several, such as production of, or ingestion of, certain acids, in such doses that the kidney and/or buffering systems cannot cope, the loss of H^+, and the loss or retention of bicarbonate. Thus, two types of both acidosis and alkalosis are recognised.

Acidosis

Acidosis (raised plasma H^+)

- Metabolic acidosis is characterised by an increased production and/or decreased excretion of H^+. Due to complex buffering with bicarbonate, levels of the latter may fall, and there may well be a compensative hyperventilation that will lead to a fall in CO_2. Examples of clinical syndromes increasing H^+ include diabetic and alcoholic ketoacidosis, lactic acidosis and poisoning by methanol, salicylate or ingestion of acids. Renal failure will lead to failure to excrete H^+ whilst bicarbonate can be lost in severe diarrhoea.

- Respiratory acidosis (raised PCO_2) is caused by an increase (probably due to retention) of CO_2. This in turn may be due to hypoventilation, itself possibly caused by drugs (e.g. narcotics, anaesthetics), nerve (motor neurone disease, poliomyelitis) or muscle problems, stroke and trauma. Respiratory diseases causing acidosis include bronchitis, asthma, fibrosis, and chronic obstructive airways disease (COAD).

Alkalosis

Alkalosis (decreased plasma H^+)

- Metabolic alkalosis (with raised bicarbonate) is often due to loss of H^+ from the gastro-intestinal tract by vomiting and diarrhoea. Certain drugs (e.g. thiazide diuretics) may cause H^+ to be lost in urine. Because ventilation is generally normal, PCO_2 levels can be unchanged (or modestly raised) and so bicarbonate rises. Another cause is excess ingestion of alkali solutions (e.g. sodium bicarbonate solution by athletes).
- Respiratory alkalosis is due to hyperventilation so that PCO_2 falls. The bicarbonate is generally normal. This may be voluntary, mechanical, or stimulation of the brain stem respiratory centre (by pain, drugs, fever, hypoxia due to high altitude, anaemia and/or pulmonary disease and oedema giving poor perfusion).

Blood sampling

Blood Sampling

Generally speaking, the greatest call for blood gases is in Accident and Emergency, Intensive Care, Neonatal Units, and in Surgery, and is often required urgently. Because of the large gradient in oxygen and carbon dioxide between venous and arterial blood, the latter is used. However, the gases in blood can exchange with those in the air so that the test must be done rapidly, and therefore the blood gas analysers are generally sited close to where they are needed although the Pathology Laboratory may also have an analyser. If blood is to be sent to the Laboratory, it should be carried rapidly in a capped, heparinised syringe, and ideally in crushed ice.

Clinical interpretation

Clinical interpretation

First, consider the H^+ level, which defines acidosis or alkalosis. Next, look at the PCO_2, and then, if necessary, the level of bicarbonate and PO_2. Interpretation can then follow.

1. Increased H^+: therefore acidosis.
   - 1.1 Decreased PCO_2, therefore metabolic acidosis. Bicarbonate is also generally reduced.
   - 1.2 Normal PCO_2, therefore uncompensated metabolic acidosis. This is likely to be because this is a simultaneous respiratory acidosis with retention of CO_2. Plasma bicarbonate will be reduced.
   - 1.3 Increased PCO_2, therefore respiratory acidosis. If this is simple, bicarbonate will be increased. However, if acute, there can be raised H^+, PCO_2 and bicarbonate (slightly) as the renal responses have yet to develop. In a chronic setting, a markedly raised bicarbonate may be present and due to renal retention.
2. Normal H^+: This does not always mean there are no metabolic problems: there may be two concurrent competing problems. For example:
   - 2.1 Decreased PCO_2, possibly because of a mixed respiratory alkalosis and metabolic acidosis. Bicarbonate is generally reduced.
   - 2.2 Normal PCO_2, therefore no acid/base disturbance.
   - 2.3 Increased PCO_2, therefore either a fully compensated respiratory acidosis, or a mixed respiratory acidosis and a concurrent metabolic alkalosis. Both lead to a raised level of bicarbonate.
3. Decreased H^+: therefore alkalosis
   - 3.1 Decreased PCO_2, therefore respiratory alkalosis. If this is uncomplicated, bicarbonate will also be decreased.
   - 3.2 Normal PCO_2, therefore uncompensated metabolic alkalosis. Plasma bicarbonate will be increased.
   - 3.3 Increased PCO_2, therefore another complex disturbance such as metabolic alkalosis with some respiration changes (i.e. hypoventilation) in compensation. Another explanation may be combined metabolic alkalosis and respiratory acidosis. Plasma bicarbonate will also be increased.

Management

Management

First, understand the aetiology and define the underlying cause. Where this is not immediately possible, then neutralisation of the pH problem should be undertaken, e.g. in metabolic acidosis, give bicarbonate slowly to buffer the H^+ if the latter exceeds 100 nmol/l (pH < 7). In respiratory acidosis the objective is to improve alveolar ventilation and so lower the PCO_2, possibly by mechanical means, or by giving oxygen. A saline drip (possibly with potassium supplementation) may be useful to stimulate renal perfusion. A common treatment for the hyperventilation of respiratory alkalosis is to get the subject to breathe into a paper bag. This will generally force more CO_2 in inspired air, and thus into the blood.

Summary of blood gases

Summary

- Arterial blood must be measured as soon as possible after it has been obtained.
- Acidosis can be respiratory (e.g. following lung disease as in COAD [chronic obstructive airways disease]) or metabolic (due to overproduction of, and/or failure to excrete H^+).
- Alkalosis can be respiratory (e.g. due to hyperventilation) or metabolic (e.g. loss of gastric secretions).

Case study 8

A woman in her mid-twenties is brought to the Accident and Emergency Unit at midnight unconscious having collapsed at a night club. Her friends do not consider her to be drunk but say she may well have hit her head as she fell. The subject is poorly responsive, pale and clammy, and with a breath rate of about 20–25/minute. Blood pressures are 110/70, pulse rate 90/minute. Serum biochemistry and blood gases are ordered.

Serum biochemistry

Na	(133–148)	150	**K**	(3.3–5.6)	3.7
Urea	(3.0–8.3)	12.2	**Creatinine**	(44–133)	85
Glucose	(< 6.1)	4.5	**Bicarbonate**	(21–28)	21

Blood gases

Hydrogen ions (H^+)	(36–44)	29	**pH**	(7.36–7.44)	7.55
Bicarbonate	(24–32)	25	**PCO_2**	(4.5–6.1)	3.8

Interpretation

The abnormal serum results are slight hypernatraemia and uraemia, with serum bicarbonate at the bottom end of the normal range. The blood pressure is not too bad but there is somewhat of a tachycardia. The blood gas result is consistent with respiratory alkalosis (raised pH, low H^+ and PCO_2, low-ish bicarbonate), which fits in with the hyperventilation (about twice the normal rate). Note the report of possible head injury that may have involved the brain stem. A check of the woman's handbag found an inhaler, implying a mild lung problem, and antibiotics, implying an unknown infection. Normal glucose rules out diabetic ketoacidosis causing the collapse. Electrolyte changes may be secondary to a pre-renal problem, possibly dehydration. Consider also the possibility of drug abuse causing a respiratory stimulation. The situation does not seem to be life threatening – the respiratory rate is not extremely high – so that rest and observation may be all that is required. A saline drip may help the pre-renal uraemia.

Chapter 13

Biochemistry Case Reports

Generally, as for the haematology, identify abnormal results, consider a primary diagnosis, and then suggest additional tests to confirm your diagnosis. Normal ranges are provided in brackets and also on page 126.

Case report 11

A 69-year-old man pops into a 'Well Man' clinic whilst out shopping with his wife. He generally considers himself to be in good health, being a non-smoker, physically active (playing golf twice a week) and is not overweight.

Na	(133–148)	138	**K**	(3.3–5.6)	3.8
Urea	(3.0–8.3)	5.3	**Creatinine**	(44––133)	92
T protein	(63–84)	69	**Albumin**	(35–50)	39
Calcium	(2.2–2.6)	2.75			
Bilirubin	(<21)	9	**Alk phosphatase**	(20–130)	145
ALT	(<41)	30	**PSA**	(<6.5)	2
Cholesterol	(2.5–5.0)	6.7	**Triglycerides**	(<2.3)	2.85
Glucose	(<6.1)	7.0	**CRP**	(<5)	1.5

Case report 12

A female, aged 75 and living alone, is admitted for investigation of intermittent abdominal pain, but is otherwise well. She has a history of pernicious anaemia. With a body mass index of 22.5 and flaking skin, she is due for a laparotomy on the 1st of December

Date	Normal range	27/11 (pre-op)	2/12	3/12	5/12
Na	(133–148)	141	151	152	143
K	(3.3–5.6)	3.4	2.7	4.9	3.6
Urea	(3.0–8.3)	6.5	6.5	3.5	3.7
Creatinine	(44–133)	63	59	66	70
T protein	(63–84)	59			
Albumin	(35–50)	36			
Calcium	(2.2–2.6)	2.17			

Case report 13

A female, aged 53 years, is married with three children. A frequent blood donor, she reported several months of general malaise when attending for a donor session. Found to be slightly anaemic, her donation was politely rejected and she was advised to visit her General Practitioner.

Na	(133–148)	136	K	(3.3–5.6)	4.8
Urea	(3.0–8.3)	11.3	Creatinine	(44–133)	354
Total protein	(63–84)	69	Albumin	(35–50)	39
Calcium	(2.2–2.6)	2.7	PTH	(7–53)	65
Free T4	(10–24)	30	TSH	(0.4–5.5)	0.2
Alanine AT	(<41)	34	Gamma GT	(<45)	33
Bilirubin	(<21)	8	Alk Phosphatase	(20–130)	112

Case report 14

A male, aged 37 years, a frequent traveller abroad, visits his family doctor with a long history of feeling generally tired and unwell, but without any precise symptoms. On examination there is tenderness on the right side of the abdomen. His diet is good, he reports no sweating or fevers, and there are no changes in his bowel habits or frequency of urination.

Na	(133–148)	136	K	(3.3–5.6)	4.9
Urea	(3.0–8.3)	6.2	Creatinine	(44–133)	101
Total protein	(63-84)	67	Albumin	(35–50)	36
Bilirubin	(<21)	25	ALT	(<41)	45
AST	(<37)	33	Alk phosphatase	(20–130)	155
Gamma GT	(<64)	154			
Calcium	(2.2–2.6)	2.4	PTH	(7–53)	20
Amylase	(< 110)	55			

Case report 15

A female, aged 59 years, reported progressive weight loss and tiredness over six to nine months. Over the last three months she also noted a growing mass in the right iliac fossa, but no pain, and even more recently was becoming 'unwell'. On examination there was also a mild splenomegaly.

Na	(133–148)	148	K	(3.3–5.6)	5.2
Urea	(3.0–8.3)	7.9	Creatinine	(44–133)	129
T protein	(63–84)	66	Albumin	(35–50)	33
Calcium	(2.2–2.6)	2.65	Bilirubin	(<21)	10
Alk phosphatase	(20–130)	706	CA 125	(0–30)	580
TSH	(0.4–5.5)	7.3	Free T4	(10–24)	4
Cholesterol	(2.5–5.0)	4.5	Triglycerides	(<2.3)	2.71

The same female, 18 months later. A blood test taken by the GP, after she complained of feeling unwell.

Na	(133–148)	139	K	(3.3–5.6)	4.1
Urea	(3.0–8.3)	3.2	Creatinine	(44–133)	103
T protein	(63–84)	61	Albumin	(35–50)	33
Calcium	(2.2–2.6)	2.45	Bilirubin	(< 21)	12
Alk phosphatase	(20–130)	90	Gamma GT	(< 45)	164
ALT	(< 41)	35	AST	(< 37)	23
Cholesterol	(2.5–5.0)	4.5	Triglycerides	(< 2.3)	2.88

Case report 16

A man of unknown age, but looking perhaps 50, is brought to Accident and Emergency by the police, having been found collapsed. He is poorly dressed, unshaven and unkempt. On examination there was no evidence of violence, concussion, or alcohol abuse, but he was thin and poorly communicative with dry lips and tongue. His pulse was 104, and his blood pressure was 95/65.

Na	(133–148)	162	K	(3.3–5.6)	4.6
Urea	(3.0–8.3)	22.9	Creatinine	(44–133)	155
T protein	(63–84)	52	Albumin	(35–50)	28
Glucose	(< 6.1)	3.0			
ALT	(< 41)	26	AST	(< 37)	30
Bilirubin	(< 21)	10	Alk Phosphatase	(20–130)	76
Gamma GT	(< 64)	45	Amylase	(< 110)	90

Case report 17

Interpret these oral glucose tolerance tests. Data are the serial levels of glucose mmol/L after the 75g of glucose taken orally.

	Time (minutes) after glucose load			
	0	**60**	**120**	**180**
1. Male, 65, obese, often tired and thirsty with some diarrhoea.	8.1	11.5	16.2	12.2
2. Male, 41, dipstick glycosuria found at a Well-Man clinic.	6.5	7.8	8.9	7.4
3. Female, 62, complains of a dry mouth and skin, and hair loss.	7.4	12.8	14.7	9.9
4. Male, 25, high fingerprick glucose at a Church fete.	4.2	6.2	6.9	5.2
5. Female, 75, high random glucose on GPs clinic machine.	6.3	7.0	7.6	6.9

Case report 18

A 55-year-old male cave explorer was trapped for 7 hours after a roof collapsed. Upon rescue, he was immediately given analgesia, and was suspected of having sustained fractures and crush injuries to the back and legs. In A&E, he was disorientated and confused with rapid breathing, a pulse of 110 and blood pressures of 100/70 mm Hg.

Na	(133–148)	151	**K**	(3.3–5.6)	6.8
Urea	(3.0–8.3)	7.9	**Creatinine**	(44–133)	137
T protein	(63–84)	72	**Albumin**	(35–50)	42
Creatine kinase	(< 150)	225	**CK - MB**	(< 25)	13
Bilirubin	(< 21)	19	**Alk phosphatase**	(20–130)	125
Gamma GT	(< 64)	54	**Glucose**	(< 6.1)	3.0

Case report 19

A 55-year-old male reports to his GP a week/10 days' history of abdominal discomfort, tiredness and loss of appetite but no fever, or other aches or pains. Following the blood sample of the 25th of October, he is admitted on the 2nd November in additional abdominal discomfort and with dark urine. These are serial bloods:

Date	25/10	8/11	15/12 (Outpatients)
Na (133–148)	142	140	141
K (3.3–5.6)	4.8	4.7	4.2
Urea (3.0–8.3)	5.4	5.6	5.6
Creatinine (44–133)	101	98	103
ALT (<41)	65	69	32
AST (<37)	49	54	26
Bilirubin (<21)	31	38	12
Alk Phosphatase (20–130)	235	412	81
Gamma GT (<64)	90	110	32
Glucose (<6.1)	4.4	n.d	
T protein (63–84)	n.d	69	
Albumin (35–50)	n.d	39	
Calcium (2.2–2.6)	n.d	2.4	
PTH (10–65)	n.d	22	
Hepatitis virus screen	n.d	negative	

n.d. = not done

Case report 20

An otherwise healthy 25-year-old female presents with progressive 24–48 hour history of malaise, headaches and nausea. In A&E, a fever, hyperventilation and tachycardia were noted, and upon further questioning she reported frequent diuresis. A full blood count was taken and a moderate neutrophil leukocytosis subsequently reported. She was admitted to a Medical Ward and blood cultures were taken. Overnight, these were found to be positive with a common bacterium. The following blood result was reported before antibiotic therapy was commenced.

Na	(133–148)	140	**K**	(3.3–5.6)	5.7
Urea	(3.0–8.3)	22.9	**Creatinine**	(44–133)	155
T protein	(63–84)	71	**Albumin**	(35–50)	42
Bilirubin	(<21)	12	**Alk phosphatase**	(20–130)	113
Gamma GT	(<45)	30	**Glucose**	(<6.1)	4.1
Bicarbonate	(21–28)	15	**CRP**	(<5)	25

Solutions to Biochemistry Case Reports

Case Report 11

Abnormal results are calcium, alkaline phosphatase, cholesterol, triglycerides and glucose. Normal LFTs and normal renal function exclude these organs as the source of raised alkaline phosphatase. Triglycerides and glucose could be raised as this is almost certainly a non-fasting sample. A repeat (fasting) test, to include PTH, is needed to confirm the abnormalities and help explain the raised calcium. A 'bone' problem may be present. The high cholesterol probably needs to be treated, initially by a 3 month trial of a low fat diet. Without blood pressure or smoking history we cannot say if this case is at a high risk of a cardiovascular event.

Case Report 12

Pre-op, U&Es are acceptable but there is low total protein and low calcium. Low total protein may be linked to this via poor diet also low in calcium. Immediately after surgery there is raised sodium and low potassium. Next day, the high sodium remains but the potassium is much improved. A few days later all is well. A number of possibilities could explain these changes, such as incorrect use of drips or a minor insult to the kidneys. It is most unlikely that the low potassium could have righted itself overnight, or may be due to the late damage of cells. More likely is an active intervention, i.e. a potassium supplement to a drip. Other aspects of the history are irrelevant. Avoid the desire to account for all such details that may be misleading.

Case Report 13

Sodium and potassium are acceptable, but there is both raised urea and raised creatinine, and the increase in creatinine is greater than the increase in urea, suggesting a chronic renal condition. Both calcium and PTH are raised, and the high T4 with low TSH suggests hyperthyroidism. Liver function tests and proteins are normal. The high creatinine is certainly a concern and demands investigation. Given the physical location of the parathyroids, the thyroid problem (which may be thyrotoxicosis) may be causing the calcium irregularities. Whether or not the renal disease and thyroid/calcium problems are linked cannot be resolved simply. The point about anaemia may be relevant as a failing kidney will produce less erythropoietin, although the definition of this anaemia is unclear.

Case Report 14

The renal profile is good but there is evidence of liver problems with several tests being abnormal. The history is suggestive of a long-term problem and questioning would have considered anything that would have provoked an acute insult. Other, more intrusive questioning may be required and supportive tests such as ultrasound would help. Differential diagnoses include poor outflow of bile from the gall bladder, perhaps due to an obstruction or maybe a tumour at the head of the bile duct, or maybe alcoholism. Certainly, a hepatitis virus screen should be done as this may indicate a low-grade infection, perhaps even chronic active hepatitis. Is the frequent foreign travel relevant?

Case Report 15

The most outstanding result is the raised CA-125 that, alongside the examination detail, is strongly suggesting of cancer of the ovary. The other abnormalities of low albumin, raised calcium and raised alkaline phosphatase may easily arise indirectly from this tumour. She also seems to be hypothyroid and with a minor hypertriglyceridaemia. Some of these problems may resolve after the surgery which would probably be quite urgent.

We presume the second sample is after this surgery, and we again find mildly low albumin but also raised gamma GT. Alkaline phosphatase and calcium are normal, but the high triglycerides remain. Annoyingly, there is no repeat CA-125 or thyroid function test. We also presume she is being treated for the latter. She may be experiencing secondaries from her ovarian cancer, and/or the effects of chemotherapy. But an alternative is drinking alcohol, known to induce a hypertriglyceridaemia as well as raised gamma GT. And after surgery for cancer of the ovary, who can blame her?

Generally, CA-125 is not fully diagnostic for ovarian cancer as it can be raised in many malignancies and some non-malignant diseases. Tumour markers are not always diagnostic but can be tools to monitor therapy. However, in this case, the large mass in the woman's lower abdomen is a strong sign.

Case Report 16

This is a reasonably clear case of dehydration where the clinical signs and laboratory tests concur. There is pre-renal uraemia, low total protein and low albumin. LFTs are acceptable and the normal glucose excludes coma linked to diabetic ketoacidosis. It looks therefore like self-neglect, possibly with malnutrition. After bed rest with rehydration, a referral to Social Services seems appropriate.

Case Report 17

- The first case is a clear diabetes mellitus: high fasting blood glucose that peaks well in excess of 11.0 and barely falls thereafter.
- The fasting glucose in the second is not that high, does not rise that much less than 11, but hardly falls. A possible diagnosis is impaired glucose tolerance.
- The third is also clear diabetes.
- The fourth should not have been tested in the first place: fasting levels are good, the response prompt and the fall also prompt. Therefore a non-diabetic picture, especially considering the circumstances of the initial fingerprick!
- The final picture features a fasting glucose that is hardly high, but the post-75g sample peaks at less than 7.8. This is suggestive of impaired fasting glycaemia.

A tentative diagnosis of diabetes needs to be confirmed by a second OGTT, and it would seem prudent to confirm other diagnoses in the same manner.

Case Report 18

With such a history, we can expect multiple abnormalities. High sodium, with high-ish urea and creatinine suggest dehydration due to water deprivation, which seems obvious with the clinical picture. The raised creatine kinase suggests damage to muscle cells, but the CK-MB within the normal range suggests that this is not of cardiac origin. Bilirubin is high-ish, and this may be due to release from damaged red blood cells, which, alongside damaged muscle cells, explains the high potassium. Low glucose may be explained by temporary starvation. Treatments include rehydration with insulin and glucose.

Case Report 19

We note that all LFTs are abnormal upon presentation (25/10) and that renal function is good. This, with the history, is presumably enough to warrant admission for further investigation (8/11) at which time all LFTs have deteriorated but proteins and albumin are normal and the hepatitis virus screen is negative. In the third sample, (15/12) all indices are normal. This case is best explained as a rapidly developing cholestasis, possibly caused by a stone in the bile duct, or infection of the gall bladder. Negative hepatitis screen rules out this possible cause. Whatever the aetiology, treatment has been successful.

Case Report 20

The history and laboratory findings (positive blood cultures, neutrophil leukocytosis) are strongly suggestive of a bacterial septicaemia. This seems to have caused the acute renal failure with the raised urea being higher than raised creatinine. Proteins, LFTs and glucose are acceptable, and raised CRP supports the inflammation. The low bicarbonate probably reflects a metabolic acidosis because of the sepsis, which could also explain the elevated potassium. Hopefully, the high dose antibiotics and plenty of fluids will do the trick.

Part Three

Combined Haematology and Biochemistry Cases

Chapter 14
Combined Case Reports

From the teaching point of view, it is convenient to treat haematology and biochemistry as separate disciplines, but there are clearly many areas where the two disciplines interact and overlap, and especially in pathology. For example, the ESR is often abnormal in thyroiditis. The following cases are illustrations where blood tests support a preliminary diagnosis. Units are omitted, and normal ranges are provided in brackets.

Case report 21

A male, aged 47 years, is on long-term dialysis for chronic (end stage) renal failure, and is virtually anuric. This routine sample was obtained just before starting on a dialysis session as he complained of feeling particularly unwell.

Biochemistry

Na	(133–148)	146	**K**	(3.3–5.6)	4.9
Urea	(3.0–8.3)	16.2	**Creatinine**	(44–133)	151
Bilirubin	(<21)	15	**ALT**	(<41)	15
AST	(<37)	23	**Alk phosphatase**	(20–130)	155
Calcium	(2.2–2.6)	2.12	**PTH**	(10–65)	25

Haematology

Haemoglobin	(13.3–16.7)	12.5	**WBCC**	(3.7–9.5)	9.1
Platelets	(143–400)	120	**Prothrombin time**	(11–14)	12
Fibrinogen	(1.5–4.0)	2.9	**ESR**	(<10)	14

Interpretation

As this case already has serious renal problems, the only questions are which of the many abnormal results are to be expected. For example, calcium is a bit low, but may be because there is no help from a failing kidney in helping to absorb this substance from the intestines. Alkaline phosphatase is high, and this may reflect renal problems, but other LFTs are acceptable.

The marginally low haemoglobin is a possible consequence of the failure of the kidney to provide sufficient erythropoietin to stimulate red cell production. The white cell count, although trending to the top of the normal range, may also be expected in this condition. However, low platelets are difficult to reconcile with this picture, but may be due to the heparin used to flush through the dialysis machine before use, thus possibly leading to heparin induced thrombocytopenia. Slightly abnormal ESR may be 'normal' in someone regularly on renal dialysis. Expert opinion is required.

Case report 22

An 89-year-old man is referred to Haematology Out-patients by his family doctor with a nine-month history of weight loss and progressive tiredness with recurrent fevers and infections that required antibiotics. He also complained of dull pain in various bones that required almost continuous analgesia.On examination he was thin and there were a few palpable lumps in the left axilla. Bloods were as follows:

Haematology

Haemoglobin	(13.3–16.7)	9.4	**WBCC**	(3.7–9.5)	14.4
Platelets	(140–400)	132	**MCH**	(27–33)	22.5
MCV	(80–98)	86.5	**MCHC**	(32–35)	32.0
Plasma viscosity	(1.5–1.72)	1.92	**ESR**	(< 10)	100

Differential:		**Absolute**	**% of the WBCC**
	Neutrophils	5.8 x 10^9/L	40.3
	Lymphocytes	7.0	48.9
	Monocytes	0.8	5.6

Differential:		Absolute	% of the WBCC
	Eosinophils	0.5	0.35
	Basophils	0.2	1.4
	Blasts	0.1	0.7

Biochemistry

Na	(133–148)	156	**K**	(3.3–5.1)	4.9
Urea	(3.0–8.3)	10.2	**Creatinine**	(44–133)	198
Bilirubin	(<21)	15	**Gamma GT**	(<64)	45
T protein	(63–84)	93	**Albumin**	(35–50)	32
AST	(<37)	33	**Alk phosphatase**	(20–130)	270
Calcium	(2.2–2.6)	3.15	**PTH**	(10–65)	5

Interpretation

There is a low haemoglobin (probably a normocytic anaemia), low platelets and a raised WBCC, mostly due to increased numbers and percentage of lymphocytes. These features suggest a leukaemia, except that the WBCC is not all that high. However, the age of the subject, alongside bone pain and a chronic presentation suggest a myeloma. The very high ESR with raised plasma viscosity both support this diagnosis. Palpable lumps (probably lymph nodes) suggest the disease is spreading out of the bone marrow, and into the blood and tissues, hence the slightly raised WBCC, which may be a plasma cell leukaemia.

The biochemistry shows a renal problem typical of a chronic condition with most LTFs, but not alkaline phosphatase, acceptable. Therefore given this picture, raised calcium is suggestive of mobilisation from bone, and the alkaline phosphatase seems to support this view. Increasing levels of calcium are likely to demand treatment with a bisphosphonate. With a very high total protein, some degree of renal impairment is likely, as confirmed with the U&E results. Thus the biochemistry strongly supports the diagnosis of advanced myeloma, although the ultimate diagnosis is with serum electrophoresis.

Case report 23

This 55-year-old woman has been in intensive care for 3 weeks with an E Coli septicaemia being treated with ciprofloxacin. Previously acidotic and developing hypotension, despite fluid support, she was placed on warfarin and briefly on LMW heparin for ?DVT. However, these were cut back because of bleeding per vagina, and gross obesity (accurate BMI impossible but estimated >35) prevented many investigations. Other problems include pyrexia (38.1˚C) and bilateral effusive sacral and buttock ulcers/sores. Psychologically she was anxious and depressed, refusing physiotherapy and the Dietician's suggestion of a naso-gastric tube. Basal crackling in both lungs was noted with respiration shallow and forced.

Haematology

PT	(11–14 secs)	19	PTT	(24–34 sec)	55
Haemoglobin	(11.8–14.8)	7.0	MCV	(80–98)	90.1
WBCC	(3.7–9.5)	20.0	Platelets	(143–400)	210
RBCC	(3.88–4.99)	2.3	Hct	(36–44)	22.6
MCH	(27.3–32.6)	30.3	MCHC	(31.6–34.9)	30.9
Fibrinogen	(1.5–4.0)	2.0			

Differential:	Cell	Numbers		Percentage
	Neutrophil	(1.7–6.1)	17.8	89.0
	Lymphocytes	(1.0–3.2)	1.00	5.0
	Monocytes	(0.2–0.6)	0.6	3.0
	Atypical cells	(0.0–0.2)	0.3	3.0

Biochemistry

Na	(133–148)	143	K	(3.3–5.6)	4.7
Urea	(3.0–8.3)	10.2	Creatinine	(44–133)	64
T protein	(63–84)	30	Albumin	(35–50)	9
Calcium	(2.2–2.6)	1.76	Gamma GT	(<45)	58
Bilirubin	(<21)	7	Alk phosphatase	(20–130)	150
AST	(<37)	63	CRP	(<5)	37
TSH	(0.4–5.5)	5.4	Free T4	(10–24)	6

Interpretation

We already know this woman is severely ill and has numerous problems. The major haematology points are the normocytic anaemia (note bleeding per vagina, low Hct and low red cell count) and marked neutrophil leukocytosis. There is also prolonged PT (due to warfarin?) and PTT (due to what?). Fortunately she has sufficient platelets and fibrinogen. Major biochemistry points are uraemia (virtually to be expected), a profoundly low albumin, and low total proteins with low calcium. High CRP is to be expected in view of the septicaemia and adds nothing of value. Other abnormalities are of minor clinical significance. Clinical history implies self-neglect and malnutrition, lung involvement, and the sores may be infected and/or a source of blood and fluid loss. She was about to have a 4-pack blood transfusion, but died the following day.

Case report 24

On the 5th of March a 57-year-old man with a diagnosis of sub-clavian thrombosis presented to the Oral Anticoagulant out-patient clinic on 3 mg warfarin daily. With an INR of 8.1 he was advised to stop taking warfarin and return on the 9th. On this date, looking unwell, a partial history of 'liver surgery for cancer' was obtained and LFTs were ordered.

Subsequently, a further history of cancer of the bowel with secondaries to the liver with partial hepatectomy one month previously was obtained from a Consultant Oncologist. Seen again on the 11th March with clear sclerotic jaundice he was referred to Liver Unit. On the 18th March he was started on 2 mg warfarin daily, and on the 23rd March, with an INR of 7.0, and being on antibiotics, his warfarin was stopped and he was referred back to the Liver Unit.

	Normal range	9th	11th	18th	23rd
Biochemistry					
Urea	(3.0–8.3)	4.5	2.7	3.5	3.2
Sodium	(133–148)	135	137	132	135
Potassium	(3.3–5.6)	4.8	4.2	5.0	4.3
Creatinine	(44–133)	71	70	63	66

	Normal range	9th	11th	18th	23rd
Albumin	(35–50)	35	34	27	28
Bilirubin	(<21)	102	133	230	197
Alk Phos	(20–130)	2772	2738	1449	4254
ALT	(<41)	730	727	164	180
Gamma GT	(<64)	1050	1149	436	1842
AFP	(<20)	3	-	2	-
Haematology					
INR	(2–3)	3.1	2.1	1.4	7.0
PTT	(24–34)	-	28.4	34.0	35.0
Fibrinogen	(1.5–4.0)	-	7.1	11.4	8.9
Haemoglobin	(13.3–16.7)	-	12.2	10.5	10.2
Haematocrit	(39–50)	-	36.7	31.3	30.6
RBCC	(4.32–5.66)	-	4.14	3.71	3.55
Platelets	(143–400)	-	448	517	535
WBCC	(3.7–9.5)	-	7.6	16.1	8.9
Neutrophils	(1.7–6.1)	-	6.1	13.9	6.9
Lymphocytes	(1.0–3.2)	-	0.64	1.1	1.5

Interpretation

This case illustrates difficulties in managing anticoagulation in patients with a rapidly failing liver, as evidenced by low albumin and rising LFTs. This is possibly due to liver secondaries, but note the low AFP. The renal picture is not that bad. However, the view of the hepatologist was of inflammatory cholestasis requiring antibiotics, a possibility supported by the neutrophil leukocytosis. Low lymphocyte numbers are just about respectable. The sudden fall in haemoglobin (2 units) may also be important and could be an internal bleed. The antibiotics interfere with warfarin, compounding the problems. Anticoagulation is certainly to be considered, even in view of the surprisingly marked hyperfibrinogenaemia and thrombocytosis with a prolonged PTT. The latter may also reflect a failing liver.

Case report 25

A 66-year-old man presents to Accident and Emergency with a short (1–2 week) history of a recently developing tiredness and lethargy. He appears thin but otherwise seemed well. The following blood result was obtained:

Haematology

PT	(11–14)	31	**PTT**	(24–34)	38
Haemoglobin	(13.3–16.7)	2.5	**MCV**	(80–98)	90
WBCC	(3.7–9.5)	656.4	**Platelets**	(143–400)	30
RBCC	(4.32–5.66)	1.85	**Hct**	(39–50)	16.6
MCH	(27.3–32.6)	22.3	**MCHC**	(31.6–34.9)	24.9

Differential:

Cell	**Normal range**	**Numbers**	**Percentage**
Neutrophils	(1.7–6.1)	72.21	11.0
Lymphocytes	(1.0–3.2)	13.13	2.0
Monocytes	(0.2–0.6)	13.13	2.0
Eosinophils	(0.03–0.46)	0	0
Basophils	(0.02–0.09)	0	0
Blasts	(~0.01)	557.93	85.0

Biochemistry

Na	(133–148)	143	**K**	(3.3–5.6)	4.3
Urea	(3.0–8.3)	5.0	**Creatinine**	(44–133)	92
Albumin	(35–50)	38	**Uric acid**	(<420)	630
ALT	(<41)	304	**Bilirubin**	(<21)	24
Alk phosphatase	(20–130)	257	**Calcium**	(2.2–2.6)	2.17
Phosphate	(0.81–1.45)	1.09	**CRP**	(<5)	51

Interpretation

With the triad of an exceptionally high WBCC, low haemoglobin and low platelets, this is clearly an acute leukaemia. High numbers of some, but absence of other, 'normal' cells are probably an artefact of the Haematology analyser – there are simply so many cells present that the machine cannot cope. Other changes are to be expected: low red cell count and haematocrit. However, there are other abnormalities – notably raised PT and PTT, as if the case were on active anticoagulation, which he was not. This may reflect the extent to which the disease has spread from the bone marrow to the liver. Remarkably, renal function seems to be unimpaired. However, there is other evidence of the disease spreading to the liver, notably raised liver enzymes. Raised CRP simply reflects very severe disease although an infection cannot be discounted.

Shortly after this report was received, the patient was due to be transferred to the leukaphoresis suite in an attempt to reduce the load of abnormal (leukaemic) cells in his blood. However, he suffered a fatal cardiac arrest whilst in transfer. The case also illustrates how rapidly this acute myeloid leukaemia developed and influenced other laboratory tests.

Appendix 1

Haematology normal values

n.b. FOR THIS BOOK ONLY – NOT FOR GENERAL USE

	Normal range
RED CELLS	
Haemoglobin (Hb)	M: 13.3–16.7, F: 11.8–14.8 g/dL
Red blood cell count (RBCC)	M: 4.32–5.66, F 3.88–4.99 x 10^{12}/L
Haematocrit (Hct)	M: 39–50%, F: 36–44%

Red cell indices

Mean cell haemoglobin (MCH)	27.3–32.6 pg
Mean cell haemoglobin concentration (MCHC)	31.6–34.9 pg/dL
Mean cell volume (MCV)	80–98 fL
Plasma viscosity	1.5–1.72 mPa
Erythrocyte sedimentation rate (ESR)	< 10 mm/hour

WHITE BLOOD CELLS

White blood cell count (WBCC) 3.7–9.5 x 10^9/L

The differential:	Absolute	Percentage
Neutrophils	1.7–6.1 x 10^9/L	40–75
Lymphocytes	1.0–3.2	20 –45
Monocytes	0.2–0.6	2–10
Eosinophils	0.03–0.46	1–6
Basophils	0.02–0.09	< 1
Blasts/atypical cells	~ 0.01	< 1

COAGULATION

Platelets	143–400 x 10^9/L
Fibrinogen	1.5–4 g/L
Prothrombin time (PT)	11–14 seconds
Partial thromboplastin time (PTT)	24–34 seconds
International normalised ratio (INR)	2–3 or 3–4

M = male, F = female

Once more, the concept of a normal range may well be restrictive and/or perjorative. For example, over the years, glucose and lipid normal ranges have fallen markedly. One may therefore describe these as reference or target ranges.

Appendix 2

Biochemistry normal values

n.b. FOR THIS BOOK ONLY–NOT FOR GENERAL USE

For convenience, the various tests are collected into various groups with a common theme.

Analyte	Unit	Normal range	Analyte	Unit	Normal range
Proteins and hormones					
Total protein	g/L	63–84	Albumin	g/L	35–50
PTH	ng/L	10–65	Free T4	pmol/L	10–24
TSH	mIU/L	0.4–5.5	CRP	mg/L	< 5
PSA	µg/L	< 6.5 (age dependent)			
Urea and electrolytes					
Calcium	mmol/L	2.2–2.6	Sodium	mmol/L	133–148
Urea	mmol/L	3.0–8.3	Potassium	mmol/L	3.3–5.6
Creatinine	µmol/L	44–133	Bicarbonate	mmol/L	21–28
Uric acid/urate	µmol/L	M < 420, F < 340	Phosphate	mmol/L	0.81–1.45
Enzymes/LFTs					
Alk Phosphatase	IU/L	20–130	Amylase	IU/L	< 110
ALT	IU/L	< 41	AST	IU/L	< 37
Gamma GT	IU/L	M < 64, F < 45	Bilirubin	µmol/L	< 21
Atherosclerosis					
Glucose	mmol/L	< 6.1	Triglycerides	mmol/L	< 2.3
Cholesterol	mmol/L	2.5–5.0	HDL-cholesterol	mmol/L	> 1.0
CK-MB	IU/L	< 25	Total CK	IU/L	< 150
HbA1c	%	3.8–6.2			
Blood Gases and pH					
Hydrogen ions (H^+)	nmol/L	36–44	pH		7.36–7.44
Bicarbonate (HCO_3^-)	mmol/L	24–32	CO_2 (PCO_2)(kPa)		4.5–6.1
Blood oxygen (PO_2)	kPa	12–15			

M = male, F = female, ALT = alanine aminotransferase,
AST = aspartate aminotransferase, CK = creatine kinase

It must AGAIN be emphasised that these values are appropriate only for this document and may not be transferable to the reader's own hospital. This is because the normal range should reflect the local population, and because different analytical methods and machines can give different results.

Appendix 3

B-type natriuretic peptide (BNP)

BNP is a relative newcomer to cardiology in general, and to heart failure in specific. Being produced by muscles of the heart wall in response to increased mechanical load and wall stretch, this molecule is gaining recognition as sensitive biomarker of cardiac dysfunction. It plays a key role in protecting the body from volume overload by maintaining renal function and sodium balance. In acute coronary syndromes increased concentrations are strong predictors of recurring myocardial infarction, heart failure, and death. BNP can also help in the assessment of the severity of ventricular dysfunction and heart failure and as a prognostic predictor, regardless of the primary cause of the condition, and can be used to guide the therapy of heart failure and left ventricular dysfunction.

BNP works best when used for specific clinical purposes, rather than for screening in the general population – its main strength is the excellent negative predictive value with regard to left ventricular dysfunction and heart failure. However, it is a non-specific biomarker of cardiac dysfunction, said by some to be a hormone, so that a specific diagnostic tool, such as ECG, is required to define an actual abnormality. For example, in dyspneic adult emergency department patients, a directed history, physical examination, chest radiograph, and electrocardiography should be performed. If the suspicion of heart failure remains, obtaining a serum BNP level may be helpful, especially for excluding heart failure.

Several well-characterised commercial assays have recently become available, but each has its own normal range. In one study, BNP levels greater than 20pg/mL were associated with significantly increased risk of heart failure and atrial fibrillation.

Further reading

I am happy to recommend the following textbooks.
They all provide considerably more information than this short work.

ABC of Clinical Haematology
Provan D and Henson A, BMJ Books, London WC1H 9JR
ISBN 0 72709 1206 2

Haematology at a Glance
Mehta A and Hoffbrand V, Blackwell Science, Oxford, 2000
ISBN 0 632 04793 3

Clinical Biochemistry
Allan Gaw et al, Churchill Livingstone, Edinburgh, 1995.
ISBN 0 443 94481 3

Clinical Biochemistry
Smith AF et al, Blackwell Science, Oxford, 1998
ISBN 0 632 04834 4

Clinical Chemistry
Marshall WJ, 4th Edition, Mosby, Edinburgh 2000
ISBN 0 7234 3159 0

Clinical Chemistry in Diagnosis and Treatment
Mayne PD. 6th Edition. Arnold, London
ISBN 0 340 57647 2

Index

Index